Auditory
Communication
for
Deaf Children

Auditory
Communication
for
Deaf Children

*A guide for teachers, parents
and health professionals*

Norman P. Erber

ACER Press

First published 2011
by ACER Press, an imprint of
Australian Council *for* Educational Research Ltd
19 Prospect Hill Road, Camberwell
Victoria, 3124, Australia

www.acerpress.com.au
sales@acer.edu.au

Edited by Diane Brown
Cover and text design by ACER Project Publishing
Typeset by ACER Project Publishing
Cover image by Jenni Ennis
Photograph on p. 72 by Norman P. Erber. All other photographs used under license from
Shutterstock.com: p. 8 © emin kuliyev; p.73 © auremar; p. 74 © Noam Armonn;
p. 78 © Martin Novak; p. 85 © Matka Wariatka; p. 142 © wavebreakmedia ltd; p. 176 © Kirill P.
Printed in Australia by BPA Print Group

National Library of Australia Cataloguing-in-Publication data:

Author:	Erber, Norman P.
Title:	Auditory communication for deaf children : a guide for teachers, parents and health professionals / Norman P. Erber.
ISBN:	9781742860206 (pbk.)
Notes:	Includes bibliographical references and index.
Subjects:	Deaf children.
	Deaf children--Language.
	Deaf children--Education.
	Deaf--Means of communication
	Hearing impaired children.
	Hearing impaired children--Education.
Dewey Number:	362.7842

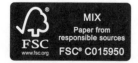

This book is printed on carbon neutral paper derived from
well-managed forests and other controlled sources certified
against Forest Stewardship Council® standards, a non-profit
organisation devoted to encouraging the responsible
management of the world's forests.

Contents

About the author

Norman P. Erber is an Associate Professor and Research Fellow at the Renwick Centre, Royal Institute for Deaf and Blind Children (Sydney, Australia). He is a clinician, research scientist, and academic with 40 years experience in the education and rehabilitation of children and adults with impaired hearing. Dr. Erber has developed many auditory assessment and therapy procedures, as well as training methods for parents and teachers, and has achieved international acclaim as the creator of the hearing-loss simulator. He is a consultant to schools, education departments, and hearing/vision-rehabilitation services. Dr. Erber has published seven textbooks and over 80 scientific articles.

Preface

The first edition of this book was called *Auditory Training* (Erber 1982). Although that popular book is now out of print, parents of hearing-impaired children, teachers, audiologists, and others continue to use many of its original concepts, including:

- an auditory skills (stimulus-response) matrix
- GASP! auditory assessment procedures
- a conversational basis for teaching and therapy
- clear speech and communication strategies
- telephone communication training methods.

This new edition updates those concepts and reviews recent progress in auditory assessment and auditory communication methods, including:

- adaptive auditory test procedures
- digital hearing aids and cochlear implants
- self-help strategies for children
- guidance for communication partners
- simulation of hearing loss.

The aims of this book are:

- to help parents, teachers, and therapists develop their interactive skills
- to help hearing-impaired children become better listeners and communicators.

The chapters contain information about speech communication, a framework for auditory assessment and therapy, and methods for providing listening experiences in a conversational context. Many listening and communication activities are included to help you adapt these methods to your needs. Practical suggestions are given on how to make auditory learning successful, what to expect, and how to maintain motivation. The reader will learn how to help a child develop auditory communication skills regardless of the listening system and instructional approach that is used.

Principles of audiology, education, language, and speech communication are presented in a simple, non-technical way. Professional jargon has been avoided where possible. A glossary provides definitions of important concepts. A pronunciation key to phonetic symbols is included (Appendix 4). Sources for related products developed by the author are provided in the back of the book.

This book does not review the research literature in detail, although it contains a large number of references to relevant publications as a guide to important source material. The ideas, methods, and materials described in this book are based mainly on my research and teaching experience at:

- Central Institute for the Deaf (St Louis, MO)
- Glendonald School for Deaf Children (Kew, VIC)
- Graduate School of Education, University of Melbourne (Parkville, VIC)
- H.E.A.R. Service (East Melbourne, VIC)
- Taralye Pre-School and Parent Advisory Centre (Blackburn, VIC)
- School of Communication Sciences, La Trobe University (Bundoora, VIC)
- Renwick Centre/Royal Institute for Deaf and Blind Children (North Rocks, NSW)

Helen O'Shea asked me to write this book. She felt there was a need to help parents, teachers, and therapists understand the process of auditory communication in everyday situations, give them the skills to help a child develop as a listener, and show them how to inform and train others.

Helen and others (Rebecca Bull, Jill Duncan, Kay Hooper, Neryl Horn, Susan Inglis, Field Rickards, Diane Toe) read earlier versions of the manuscript and provided direction regarding its content and accuracy.

Lois MacCullagh, an experienced medical writer and editor, read later versions of the manuscript, suggested changes in organization, and gave the text clarity.

For Sophie

"Listen:…
…Poo-tee-weet?"

Kurt Vonnegut (*Slaughterhouse Five*, 1969)

CHAPTER 1

Introduction

Much has changed in the fields of audiology, hearing technology, and parental guidance since the first edition of this book was published more than 25 years ago. Significant advances include the following:

- audiologists can identify hearing impairments in infants with a high degree of accuracy
- programmable hearing aids and cochlear implants are available to very young hearing-impaired children
- parents are recognized as major contributors to their child's development of spoken language.

Educators agree that a child's hearing and hearing aids/cochlear implants are important factors in acquisition of speech and language. Some educators promote an auditory approach, in which visible cues for speech are minimized and acoustic cues are emphasized (Estabrooks 2006). Others encourage the child to simultaneously look and listen to maximize speech input during daily conversation (Simmons-Martin & Rossi 1990). Regardless of method, the aim is to help the child establish an auditory foundation for reception and expression of spoken language similar to that used by children with normal hearing. Research has shown that many hearing-impaired children who received meaningful listening experiences from infancy have developed communication skills in parallel with their hearing peers (Rhoades & Chisholm 2000; Geers et al., 2003b; Dornan et al., 2010; Geers et al., 2011).

HUMAN INTERACTION

When a child is very young, most social exchange is with members of the family. As the child grows and matures, however, there is more contact with friends, neighbors, and others in the community. The child learns to interact in several ways including:

- awareness of other people
- expression of emotional states

1

- declaration of wants and needs
- requesting, giving, and getting information
- development of goal-oriented relationships
- development of friendships and social relationships.

Building relationships requires life experience, maturity, and the ability to participate in conversation. Conversation requires auditory perception and communication of spoken language.

Perception

Auditory perception is an essential component of speech communication. Auditory perception involves awareness, decoding, and interpretation of sounds. In most social interaction, the sounds are *speech* sounds. Auditory perception of speech is a complex process that begins in the child's ears and ends in the child's brain.

Children perceive what people say and do mainly through vision, touch, and hearing. We can observe where a child looks and what a child touches, but we cannot easily observe what a child *hears*. Auditory perception of speech can only be inferred by observing the child's responses at several different levels: detection, discrimination, recognition, and comprehension. In some cases, an auditory response is a natural reflex (the child looks when someone speaks). In other cases, the response has been *learned* (the child points to a picture of an elephant when someone speaks the word *elephant*).

Development of the hearing-impaired child's auditory perception is a primary focus of daily communication. One approach is to speak with the young child in a natural manner during all activities, with an expectation for normal acquisition of listening skills and spoken language. At other times, the adult may provide practice on specific aspects of auditory perception.

Communication

Communication is the act of sending messages and their meanings from one person to another (Levinson 1983). When someone speaks, that person may express a greeting, make a request, ask a question, describe an experience, present an opinion, or share a feeling/emotion. When another person receives this message, communication has occurred.

For a hearing-impaired child, successful speech communication depends on many factors. It may require:

- a meaningful situation and context
- a clearly articulated message
- a quiet and non-distracting environment
- an appropriate personal listening system
- the child's attention to the task.

Conversation

Conversation is a form of social interaction in which people use language in a systematic, reciprocal manner. A conversation occurs when two or more people exchange opinions, thoughts, or feelings according to socially accepted procedures. People converse for many reasons – to form and maintain friendships, acquire empathy, gain insight, and influence others. The outcome of a conversation may be a new, shared point of view (Wardhaugh 1985; Myllyniemi 1986).

Most conversations between people with normal hearing are conveyed through spoken language and involve the production and perception of *speech*. An important goal for a hearing-impaired child is the ability to engage in conversation through speech (Tye-Murray 1994, 2003).

A *fluent* conversation is an exchange of talk without confusion, long silences, or domination by one of the participants. A smooth flow of conversation depends on the auditory and visual intelligibility of the messages, knowledge of spoken language, and awareness of the social structure of human interaction.

As hearing-impaired children develop conversational skills, they and their communication partners may experience misunderstandings. Resolution of a conversational difficulty usually requires:

- awareness of the difficulty
- a clarification request
- a clarification strategy
- successful repair
- restoration of conversational flow.

HISTORY OF AUDITORY (RE)HABILITATION

Auditory (re)habilitation is a term used to describe the creation of a listening and learning environment in which parents, teachers, and therapists help children with impaired hearing to acquire speech communication skills. To many audiologists and educators, the process consists of obtaining audiometric information, providing appropriate hearing aids or cochlear implants, maintaining the child's personal listening system, and communicating through speech. Some hearing-impaired children are able to develop auditory communication skills when parents and teachers simply establish these basic listening and learning conditions.

In many cases, however, sustained auditory progress requires the persistent efforts of parents, teachers, and therapists who provide listening experiences for the child – not only incidentally but also consciously and carefully. These adults create optimal listening conditions and help the child develop auditory abilities beyond those that might be achieved without such involvement.

Many scientists and educators have contributed to current practices in auditory habilitation for children. Significant advances in hearing technology have also occurred. This section describes the background of the methods employed by teachers and clinicians today and provides references the reader can consult for more information. This brief historical review is presented in approximate chronological order.

Auditory training

In Vienna in the late 19th century, Victor Urbantschitsch (1895) practiced systematic "auditory training" with hearing-impaired children. He demonstrated that children who appeared unresponsive to sound when first tested could improve their listening performance after concentrated instruction and practice. Many children progressed from differentiation of vowels to perception of complete sentences. He convinced other educators that auditory training was an effective instructional method.

Vibro-tactile aids

In the 1920s and 30s, before the development of practical electrical hearing aids, Robert Gault and his colleagues at Northwestern University (Evanston, IL), developed a simple vibro-tactile aid that allowed deaf people to acquire information about intensity patterns in speech. Gault and his colleagues collected information about the sensory capabilities of the skin as a speech receptor. With practice, a person could learn to make increasingly finer distinctions among speech patterns. Many deaf participants learned to distinguish sentences in limited sets, locate stress in words and sentences, and even identify or classify individual vowels and consonants (Gault 1927, 1930, 1936).

Gault demonstrated that the intensity pattern cues from a vibro-tactile aid could benefit deaf people. They typically identified spoken words and sentences better when they lipread with a vibro-tactile device than when they used lipreading alone (Gault 1927). Gault's work led to the later development of multi-channel vibro-tactile aids (Summers 1992; Galvin et al., 2001).

The acoustic method

In the 1930s and 40s, Max Goldstein, the founder of Central Institute for the Deaf (St. Louis, MO), popularized the "acoustic method", an approach to auditory learning derived from the work of Urbantschitsch (1895). He stressed the need for daily stimulation of the hearing-impaired child's auditory system (Goldstein 1939). He claimed that all children, regardless of the severity of the hearing loss, could benefit from experience in perceiving acoustic cues for speech. He also demonstrated the importance of auditory feedback to speech development.

Goldstein created a variety of listening exercises, which included vowel perception, syllable drills, and identification of words and sentences. He promoted the use of the first electrical hearing aids. Goldstein devoted considerable energy to convincing the medical profession of the auditory potential of hearing-impaired children, especially the role that *listening* could play in their development of spoken language.

Wired classroom hearing aids

In the 1940s and 50s, Clarence Hudgins at the Clarke School for the Deaf (Northampton, MA) evaluated some of the first wired classroom (group) hearing aids (Hudgins 1948, 1954). He demonstrated that regardless of the amount of hearing loss, children with impaired hearing could benefit from listening to speech at appropriately amplified levels. He showed that listening practice could increase word understanding, as well as improve speech and academic progress. Hudgins confirmed Gault's notion that even profoundly deaf children could learn to use the amplified sounds of speech to aid lipreading (Hudgins 1954). These findings encouraged other educators to use hearing aids in their classrooms. Moreover, Hudgins' results raised expectations for successful speech communication in all hearing-impaired children.

The auditory-oral method

In the 1950s and 60s, several versions of the "Auditory-Oral" method emerged. These versions were applied and promoted by Wedenberg (1951, 1954), Ewing and Ewing (1961), van Uden (1970), and Simmons (1971). These educators strongly advocated early detection of hearing loss. The use of carefully selected and adjusted hearing aids was considered a major factor in the auditory development of the young hearing-impaired child. An important component of this method was active participation by *parents* in their child's learning and communication development. This method departed from earlier acoustic methods in two ways: (1) the child was encouraged to look and listen most of the time and (2) the method was based on a natural development of speech and language skills, rather than the more analytical teaching procedures employed by earlier educators.

Amplification systems and strategies

In the 1960s and 70s, manufacturers began to produce miniature hearing aid microphones and circuitry. Small hearing aids and earmolds were created specifically for use by children. New approaches to amplification emerged. Some educators advocated increased attention to a child's low-frequency hearing and greater amplification of speech sounds in that frequency range. Guberina (1964), Ling (1964), and Asp (1973) reported positive results in speech perception and production by extending amplification into the lower frequencies.

The "verbotonal system" (Guberina 1964) employed selective amplification in "optimal" frequency regions, vibro-tactile aids, rhythmic speech instruction, and special attention to intonation and stress patterns in developing the receptive and expressive language of young hearing-impaired children. Concentrated listening practice with individual children was considered an important contributor to success.

New technology was developed to modify the amplified speech signal. For example, Johansson (1966) introduced the transposer hearing aid, which electronically shifted high-frequency speech energy to a lower frequency range. Others also have described the potential benefits of frequency transposition to hearing-impaired children (Auriemmo et al., 2009; Glista et al., 2009).

In the 1970s, manufacturers began to develop high-quality, miniature behind-the-ear hearing aids, usually worn binaurally. Children's amplification systems became smaller and lighter.

Wireless amplification systems were produced that used electromagnetic induction, FM transmission, or infrared radiation to transmit speech energy at a distance from the speaker to the child (Madell 1992; Ross 1992; Compton 2000). More recently, sound-field amplification systems have been introduced for use in classrooms and other large areas (Crandell et al., 2005). All these amplification systems increase mobility, encourage natural interaction between the child and others, and improve communication in moderately noisy environments.

Digital hearing aids

Digital signal processing in hearing aids now permits modification of frequency response and amplification characteristics to match each child's requirements for louder sound and listening comfort. Computer-based hearing aid selection procedures specify an optimal hearing aid output for each child's hearing loss (Dillon 2001; Seewald et al., 2005). Software is available to automatically adapt the aid's characteristics to environmental conditions and to minimize effects of noise. Directional microphones enable emphasis of the speaker's voice and suppression of unwanted noises. Fast-acting filters are used to eliminate feedback squeal (Harkins & Bakke 2003).

Electrophysiological tests of hearing

Auditory Brainstem Response (ABR) and Auditory Steady State Response (ASSR) are electrophysiological test methods that audiologists use to measure hearing loss in infants and young children who cannot provide behavioral responses. In each method, several electrodes are placed on the child's head. Acoustic clicks (ABR) or tones of changing quality (ASSR) are presented through miniature earphones placed in the ear canals. The brain's responses to sounds are amplified and recorded by a computer. Careful examination of the data yield an accurate estimate of the child's hearing sensitivity (Stapells 2000; Rance 2008). These test methods also can be used to assess the benefit of amplification for infants.

Cochlear implants

A cochlear implant is an electronic device designed to restore auditory sensation and perception to a child with a significant hearing loss. Sound is detected by a miniature microphone, encoded by a small digital signal processor, and presented as electrical pulses to multiple electrodes surgically implanted in the child's inner ear. Cochlear implants are available to children with severe to profound hearing impairments who have experienced little progress in auditory communication with hearing aids, and whose family strongly support the child's auditory development. An implant typically produces an "aided threshold" in the range 20–40 dB HL (decibels Hearing Level), and permits detection of most speech sounds at a conversational level.

Speech perception differs among children who have received implants (Gstoettner et al., 2000). The differences are attributed to variations in cochlear anatomy and physiology, quality of nerve transmission between the ear and the brain, duration of deafness, previous listening experience, communication mode, age at implantation, speech processing strategy, and duration of implant use (Sarant et al., 2001; Spencer & Marschark 2003; Geers 2006; Nicholas & Geers 2006). According to many researchers, a typical outcome is development of auditory communication skills similar to those of a child with a pure tone hearing loss between about 60 and 90 dB HL who has used hearing aids (i.e., a child with a moderate-to-severe hearing impairment) (Boothroyd et al., 1991; Boothroyd & Eran 1994; Vermeulen et al., 1997; Meyer et al., 1998; Blamey & Sarant 2002; Rotteveel et al., 2008).

The auditory-verbal method

Early identification of hearing loss in children, and improvements in amplification and cochlear implant technology led to a major shift in educational emphasis in the 1970s and 80s. Unisensory ("acoupedic") instruction as previously advocated by Beebe (1953), Griffiths (1967), and Pollack (1970, 1984) gained prominence. This method, now called "auditory-verbal", has retained strong support from a dedicated group of therapists. Features of auditory-verbal practice include:
- early detection of hearing loss
- early application of hearing aids/cochlear implants
- parent training

- one-to-one instruction
- reduction of visible cues for speech
- frequent assessment of auditory progress
- early integration into regular school.

The aim of this method is to help children reach their potential as *auditory* communicators. Parents and therapists provide both natural conversation and planned listening activities. To encourage listening, the adult positions herself near the child. Together, they may participate in a play activity or learning task (see figure 1.1). Visual attention to the mouth is not encouraged.

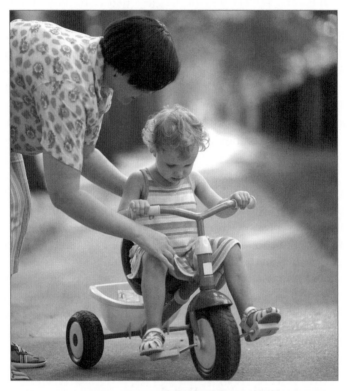

Figure 1.1 **A mother communicates with her child during play**

From birth to five years, the child receives a variety of auditory experiences in a good environment (one-to-one interaction; near distance; in a quiet location). Later, the child learns to listen in small groups and with background noise. Individual instruction is recommended for most listening practice. In everyday situations and environments, the child is helped to develop listening skills, an auditory feedback mechanism for speech, and natural spoken language.

A principal goal is integration into a school for children with normal hearing, where the child is taught by a classroom teacher, who may be assisted by an auditory therapist. In a classroom, the learning environment may not be optimal (greater distance, noise, and distraction), and so specific listening skills are taught to help the child learn in the same environment as hearing peers.

CURRENT PRACTICES

A large amount of research now is directed to early diagnosis of hearing impairment and appropriate fitting of personal listening systems to infants and young children. Audiologists are routinely involved with the selection, programming, and maintenance of hearing aids and/or cochlear implants. In many educational settings for hearing-impaired children, considerable attention is directed to the auditory components of communication. Parents, therapists, and teachers devote much of their time to helping the child learn to perceive and produce speech. The principal aims are age-appropriate language skills, conversational competence, and academic progress (Geers & Hayes 2011; Geers & Sedey 2011).

SUMMARY

A young hearing-impaired child must learn to listen and interpret the sounds that are received through hearing aids and/or cochlear implants. Natural interaction in meaningful situations and directed listening practice are essential to the child's progress as a communicator. Informed parents are recognized as major contributors to the child's development of spoken language.

CHAPTER 2

Speech perception

The rate at which a hearing-impaired child develops spoken language is related to the child's ability to perceive speech (O'Donoghue et al., 1999; Lachs et al., 2001). This chapter provides a broad description of the perceptual capabilities and limitations of children with various degrees of hearing impairment. It summarizes the results of many research studies and observations in classrooms and clinics.

This chapter is not intended to describe a specific hearing-impaired child's listening skills or potential for auditory learning. The ease with which a child learns to perceive and produce speech is influenced not only by hearing capacity, but also by hearing aids/cochlear implants, the clarity and creativity of communication partners, the acoustic environment, and the situation in which communication occurs.

To learn to listen and communicate through spoken language, the child must develop a satisfactory method for perceiving speech and monitoring/controlling speech. In particular situations, some acoustic components of speech may not be audible, or may be heard without clarity. A parent, teacher, or therapist can help by providing regular opportunities for listening and practice in recognizing minimal acoustic cues (Erber 1982; Pollack 1984; Srinivasan 1996; Easterbrooks & Estes 2007; Romanik 2008). The child can learn to identify a spoken message by combining situational, contextual, linguistic, and visible information with the cues that are received through hearing.

AUDITORY PERCEPTION

A child with a sensori-neural hearing impairment does not simply hear speech sounds as weaker than normal, as would result from a blockage of the ear canal. Instead, even when listening carefully through hearing aids or cochlear implants, the child hears various sound qualities of speech differently from how a person with normal hearing would hear them (Summerfield 1987). The child may hear some speech sounds at a reduced volume, or not at all. Some speech sounds may be distorted in quality. Some syllables and words that normally would be distinguished easily, for example, may not be heard clearly and may sound similar.

Suprasegmental patterns

The "suprasegmental" patterns of speech include changes in the intensity, duration, and/or pitch of a speaker's voice during articulation of a word, phrase, or sentence. These factors contribute to rhythm, stress, or intonation. In English, words differ with regard to the number of syllables and syllable pattern (e.g., *cat, cattle, catfish, caterpillar*). The acoustic stress pattern of a word is an important part of its identity.

A speaker may use rhythm, stress, and/or intonation to emphasize important words in order to convey the meaning of a sentence. For example, a person may stress a word in a sentence by increasing its intensity and duration ("That's *my* pen!"). A rising voice pitch may be used to indicate that a spoken sentence is not a statement, but rather a question ("Her birthday is *today*?"). A speaker may use complex changes in the voice to convey emotion and/or intent (anger, surprise, pleasure).

Most hearing-impaired children can learn to recognize intensity changes in speech. In general, children with mild-to-severe hearing impairments can identify not only intensity cues, but also intonation and melody (Most & Peled 2007). Their ability to extract meaning from this information, however, depends on instruction and listening experience (Klieve & Jeanes 2001). A child with poorer hearing may be able to recognize variations in speech intensity through hearing aids, but perhaps not variations in voice pitch. Cochlear implants may make the pitch patterns more accessible.

Intensity cues

The individual ("segmental") sounds of speech differ in their intensities and frequencies. Vowels that are produced with an open vocal tract (e.g., /ɑ/ or /ɔ/) have greater intensity than vowels that are produced with a smaller sound channel (e.g., /i/ or /u/). Some consonants (e.g., the low frequency nasal /n/) are moderately strong, but other consonants (e.g., the high frequency fricative /f/) are much weaker. Children with *normal* hearing can detect all of the speech sounds of their language when someone speaks these sounds in a normal voice at a conversational distance. A hearing-impaired child, however, may be unable to detect some of the sounds of speech. Even when listening through hearing aids or cochlear implants, the child may be unable to detect particular speech sounds if the speaker is too far away, speaks with a soft voice, or produces the speech sounds in a weak syllable.

Frequency cues

Auditory perception of speech also depends on the ability to hear small differences between sound frequencies (e.g., /m/ vs /n/ or /ʃ/ vs /s/). A child's ability to recognize familiar words is related to the ability to discriminate frequencies (Risberg et al., 1975; Ochs et al., 1989).

The frequency discrimination abilities of hearing-impaired children are often poorer than those of children with normal hearing (Risberg et al., 1975). We may think of poor frequency discrimination as a type of auditory distortion, where the sound quality of a tone is heard without clarity, and appears similar to the sound quality of other tones.

An "audiogram" is a graph that describes the softest tone a child can detect (in dB HL) at each of several test frequencies (in Hertz, or Hz). For most children with "mild" to "moderate" impairment (i.e., hearing thresholds from about 30 to 60 dB), the ability to distinguish frequencies is almost normal. These children can discriminate between two tones that differ by about 1 to 2 per cent (in Hz). For children with "severe" impairment (i.e., hearing thresholds from about 70 to 90 dB), however, there are large individual differences in frequency discrimination, ranging from about 2 to 30 per cent (i.e., from nearly normal to poor). For children with "profound" impairment (i.e., hearing thresholds greater than about 100 dB), frequency discrimination generally is very poor. These children require a 5 to 40 per cent difference in frequency in order to distinguish tones (Risberg et al., 1975).

Auditory neuropathy spectrum disorder (ANSD) is a condition that reduces the quality of information transmitted from the ear to the brain (Berlin et al., 2007). This condition is present in about 10 to 15 per cent of hearing-impaired children. ANSD can affect a child's perception of details in the frequency and timing of speech sounds. Many children with ANSD have difficulty distinguishing sounds and do not hear speech clearly, especially in background noise.

Perceptual experiences

Some perceptual experiences of children with hearing-impairment are that, typically:
- they cannot hear weak sounds without hearing aids or cochlear implants
- they can hear better in some frequency ranges than others
- they hear some sounds without clarity, even if the sounds are made louder and more audible.

Vowel perception

Vowel sounds are produced when air exhaled by the speaker's lungs passes through the larynx, causing the vocal folds to vibrate at the "fundamental" voice frequency.

The rhythmic pulses of air produced by the larynx flow through the throat, mouth, and nose cavities. The dimensions of these cavities determine which frequencies are resonated and therefore made stronger. The shape of the mouth cavity is related to the positioning of the tongue and lips, which create the distinctive sound qualities of each spoken vowel.

Each vowel contains concentrations of resonant sound energy in narrow frequency ranges called "formants". Children with normal hearing identify vowels mainly from sound energy in the lowest two formants – typically within the frequency range from 250 to 2500 Hz (see figure 2.1). A hearing-impaired child may misperceive these sounds, however, and confuse vowels that have similar formant frequencies. For example, the child might identify the spoken vowel /ɪ/ as /i/ or /ɛ/, and confuse the words *bit*, *beet*, and *bet*.

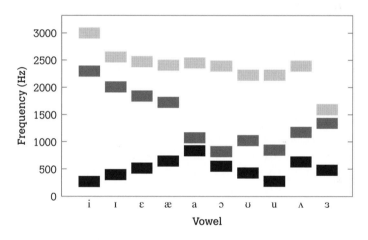

Figure 2.1 **Formant frequencies of some English vowels**

Some vowels have a similar low-frequency first formant (F1) and differ mainly in the frequency of the second formant (F2), such as the vowels /i/ and /u/ in the words *beet* and *boot*. A child who cannot clearly perceive F2 is likely to confuse these vowels, so the words *beet* and *boot* will therefore sound similar.

During a speech perception test, children respond differently when they are uncertain about what they have heard (e.g., *beet* or *boot*?). Some choose randomly between these words, but others show a clear preference for one of them (perhaps the more familiar one, or the one whose vowel contains the lower second formant). Some children not only confuse vowels produced with similar sound qualities (/i/, /ɪ/, and /ɛ/) but also confuse vowels with similar first formants (/ɪ/ and /U/). Therefore, when they listen to a word that contains the vowel /ɪ/ (e.g., *pit*), they may hear the vowel as /i/ or /ɛ/ or even as /U/, and thus identify the word *pit* as *Pete*, *pet*, or *put* (Hack & Erber 1982; Valimaa et al., 2002a).

A diphthong is a vowel that changes in sound quality (e.g., as in the words *cake, toy, hide, cow, boat*). A diphthong is produced by a smooth transition from one tongue position to another, with a corresponding change in the sound of the resonant (formant) frequencies. Hearing-impaired children may have difficulty identifying one or both components of a diphthong.

Consonant perception

Consonants are produced in different ways, for example:

- fricative – the vocal tract is constricted; exhaled air (with or without vibration from the larynx) flows through this narrow aperture and produces a noisy, continuous sound (e.g., /f, θ, ʃ, s, v, ð, ʒ, z/)
- nasal – the vocal tract is closed by the lips or tongue tip/base; the velum (soft palate) is lowered and vibrating air from the larynx flows through the nose cavity (e.g., /m, n, ŋ/)
- lateral/liquid/semivowel – vibrating air from the larynx is diverted around or over the tongue through a narrowed vocal tract, producing a "vowel-like" sound (e.g., /l, r, w, j/)
- stop/plosive – exhaled air flows through the vocal tract; the passage is closed briefly by the lips or tongue tip/base, and then is opened suddenly, permitting the air to flow again (e.g., /p, t, k, b, d, g/)
- affricate – the vocal tract is closed as for a stop/plosive consonant, but the passage does not open suddenly; instead, the air is released slowly through a fricative-like constriction (e.g., /tʃ, dʒ/).

The stop/plosive consonants are particularly difficult for hearing-impaired children to distinguish and identify. The main reason is that these consonants are not continuous sounds, but they are spoken rapidly and in close association with a preceding or following vowel. They consist of three parts: closure of the vocal tract, build-up of pressure, and sudden release of air-flow. Voiced stops (/b, d, g/) are produced with laryngeal vibration *before* the moment of release. Voiceless stops (/p, t, k/) are produced with a noisy aspiration of air *after* release and before laryngeal vibration resumes. A shift in the resonant (formant) frequencies of adjacent vowels results from rapid changes in the shape of the vocal tract during closure and release. Each of these events produces important acoustic cues for differentiation of stop/plosives. Some children have difficulty hearing the noisy burst of an unvoiced stop/plosive (as in /p, t, k/), or details in the rapid formant transitions of adjacent vowels.

Children with mild-to-severe hearing impairments usually can learn to distinguish among types of consonants that have very different sound qualities: unvoiced stops (/p, t, k/), voiced stops (/b, d, g/), unvoiced fricatives (/f, θ, ʃ, s/), voiced fricatives (/v, ð, ʒ, z/), nasals (/m, n, ŋ/), and laterals/liquids/semivowels (/l, r, w, j/) (Boothroyd 1984, 1991; Valimaa et al., 2002b) (see figure 2.2). When children can hear the differences between these consonant categories, they can distinguish between the words *pat, bat, sat, that, mat*, and *rat*. These children, however, may not hear differences among consonants within categories, and thus confuse the words *fin, thin, shin*, and *sin* – all of which begin with unvoiced fricatives.

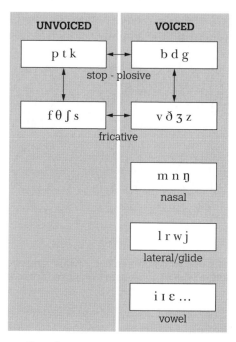

Figure 2.2 **Auditory perception of consonants. Commonly confused consonants appear in boxes. Arrows between boxes indicate confusions between consonant types**

Some children with mild-to-severe hearing impairments confuse unvoiced stop/plosives and unvoiced fricatives (e.g., *get* < > *guess*), and also confuse voiced stop/plosives and voiced fricatives (e.g., *boat* <> *vote*) (Valimaa et al., 2002b). Many hearing-impaired children can distinguish between nasal and non-nasal consonants (Erber 1972a). When a nasal consonant (/m, n/) is misidentified, it may be confused with a lateral/liquid/semivowel (/r, l, w, j/) (Valimaa et al., 2002b). Laterals/liquids/semivowels are confused occasionally with vowels that have similar low-frequency sound energy. Words that contain more than one consonant in the group of "low-frequency continuants" (/m, n, l, r, w, j/) tend to be difficult for some children to identify, especially when these speech sounds occur in a central position between two syllables (e.g., as in the words *money, always, silly, woman*).

A child with poor frequency discrimination skills can usually perceive changes in speech *intensity* (Boothroyd 1984). The child would probably be able to distinguish a voiced stop/plosive consonant from a voiced continuant in a central position, as the stop/plosive is characterized by a break in the syllable pattern, but the continuant is not characterized in this way (see figure 2.3). The same child may not be able to recognize initial or final consonants in single words, however. For example, in the word *cat* (/kæt/) the high-frequency bursts of sound energy in unvoiced /k/ and /t/ are weak, and produce little change in intensity before or after the vowel. Thus, a child with a profound hearing impairment might not be able to distinguish between the word /kæt/ and /æ/ alone – unless the child listens with a cochlear implant, which usually increases the audibility of high-frequency consonants.

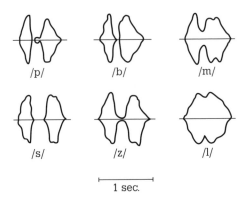

Figure 2.3 **Intensity of sound between two vowels can provide information about the type of consonant produced (Erber 1982)**

In some contexts, nasals and laterals/liquids/semivowels may be identified as a distinct consonant group because of the slow rise and fall of their intensity patterns. Some children with poor hearing can learn to use this cue to distinguish the acoustic pattern for *man* from the pattern for *bat*, or *muddy* from *money*.

Word identification

Audiologists typically assess a child's hearing for speech with lists of one-syllable words. A child may perceive some words accurately, but perceive others with greater difficulty. Some common auditory errors are shown in table 2.1.

Table 2.1 **Examples of error responses to one-syllable words by hearing-impaired children**

mats > mat	final consonant deletion
tea > teeth	final consonant addition
mouth > mouse	unvoiced fricative substitution
days > Dave	voiced fricative substitution
whip > wit	unvoiced stop substitution
door > bore	voiced stop substitution

Table 2.1 **continued**

bed > pet	voiced-unvoiced stop substitution
buzz > bus	voiced-unvoiced fricative substitution
stick > sick	unvoiced consonant blend reduction
broom > room	voiced consonant blend reduction
meat > neat	nasal consonant substitution
clown > crown	lateral/liquid consonant substitution
tick > took	vowel formant F2 inaudible
ship > sheep	vowel formants F1 and F2 misperceived

Experience suggests that a hearing-impaired child will be able to identify a spoken word more easily through listening alone if the word:
- contains a strong vowel (e.g., *dog*)
- begins with a low-frequency consonant (e.g., *mat*)
- begins with a voiced consonant (e.g., *zoo*)
- contains more than one syllable (e.g., *doctor*)
- contains more than one stressed syllable (e.g., *football*)
- contains medial consonants that are not continuants (e.g., *meeting*, but not *meaning*)
- contains no consonant blends (e.g., *team*, but not *steamed*)
- is a familiar word (e.g., *water*). Some common words such as *cake* and *cat*, however, are difficult to identify because they are short and begin/end with high-frequency consonants.

Sentence identification

Sentences also differ in ease of identification based on their acoustic characteristics, length, and complexity. Experience suggests that, in general, hearing-impaired children can identify a spoken sentence more easily through listening if the sentence:
- contains relatively few words
- contains simple syntax (e.g., subject-verb-object-prepositional phrase), without embedded clauses
- contains an animate subject (e.g., *man, nurse, cat*)
- contains an active verb (e.g., *found, gave, scratched*)
- contains no negatives (e.g., *not*)
- contains no contractions (e.g., *he's*)
- is not a yes/no question (e.g., "Is it a …?")
- is redundant/predictive (e.g., "The boy kicked the football.")
- contains common, familiar words.

PERCEPTION AND SPEECH MONITORING

Many hearing-impaired children learn to produce acoustically intelligible speech in spite of their auditory limitations (Ling 1989). Over the years, a variety of instruments and instructional techniques have been developed to help children recognize and produce acceptable speech patterns and sound qualities.

Some techniques that rely on *acoustic* cues include:

- amplifying the sounds of speech through hearing aids (Beebe 1953; Griffiths 1967; Pollack 1970; Ling 1976)
- modifying the sounds of speech through hearing aids or cochlear implants with the aim of matching the acoustic signal to the child's impaired auditory system – e.g., multi-band compression, frequency transposition, digital signal processing (Dillon 2001)
- using the sounds of speech to model/guide/reinforce the child's use of spoken language.

Some techniques that rely on *visible* cues include:

- modeling the production of mouth shapes, tongue positions, and facial expressions
- using visible hand cues ("phonetic signs") to supplement unavailable articulatory features (Schulte 1978)
- using special electronic devices to detect and display a visible pattern of speech features such as voicing, nasality, or articulation (Bernstein et al., 1988; Dagenais et al., 1994)
- guiding/reinforcing the child's use of clear speech with a nod, smile, or gesture (Calvert & Silverman 1975).

The compensatory methods listed above are intended to help the child judge the correctness of his/her own speech, and thus recognize and produce speech that will be intelligible to people with normal hearing. To transfer this ability to everyday conversation, the child must eventually learn to substitute a personal feedback system and self-judgment for special external stimulation, information, instruction, or prompting previously relied on. One function of hearing aids and cochlear implants is to continuously provide this type of personal auditory feedback.

Both normal-hearing and hearing-impaired children typically learn to produce speech through perception and imitation of an adult's speech. Teachers apply instructional strategies that formalize and/or systematize this demonstration-perception-imitation approach. They consider the child's sensory capacity in the primary mode (e.g., hearing) and rely on this mode where possible, but also devise ways that secondary modes (vision, tactile senses) can support speech and language learning. To perceive speech and develop spoken language as the result of daily interaction with parents, siblings, and teachers, the child must effectively use all available sensory information.

The best way for children to learn to produce the sounds of speech is through hearing, but first it is necessary to ensure that they can perceive the sounds. In one prescriptive method (Ling & Ling 1978: Ling 1989), a teacher or therapist assesses the child's perceptual abilities through the various sensory systems and provides speech models in a specified sequence: auditory, auditory-visual, visual (alone), and visual-tactile. If *hearing* is adequate, *acoustic* models will be sufficient, and the child will learn to match speech production to model utterances, even though the mouth cannot be seen (Beebe 1953; Pollack 1970). It can be difficult, however, to teach some speech features to some children through hearing alone, because auditory perception is insufficient. In these instances, visible articulation or tactile feedback may be helpful. After the child acquires the speech feature, the acoustic model alone may be used to reinforce learning.

Speech perception and production are often taught simultaneously through modeling and imitation. The following sequence is employed:

1 demonstrate correct production of a sound, word, phrase, or sentence through listening alone
2 the child perceives your spoken model
3 the child imitates your model
4 the child perceives his/her own vocal output
5 the child compares his/her imitation with (memory of) your utterance
6 the child judges the similarity/correctness of the imitation.

Development of speech through imitation requires the child to perceive both your model and his/her own utterance. It is not possible to directly observe the child's speech perception process, however, and thus judge its accuracy. But you can observe the behavioral consequences of a child's perception.

It may be appropriate to teach and assess *perception* (depending on the age of the child). The following steps are recommended:

1 you show the child a set of pictures (e.g., *coat, goat*)
2 you associate a spoken stimulus (word) with each picture
3 you ask the child to listen
4 you speak one of the words ("coat")
5 you ask the child to choose among the alternatives
6 the child responds by pointing to his or her choice
7 you reward a correct response; you acknowledge (or ignore) an incorrect response.

If the child responds correctly most of the time, you can infer that the desired auditory perception has occurred (i.e., the child can hear what you said). If incorrect responses are common, however, you can conclude that either the child is experiencing perceptual difficulty, or you have incorrectly explained or presented the task. With practice, you should be able to create and present listening tasks in such a way that the child is fully aware of, and can focus on, the particular feature or detail. During instruction, you may vary stimulus and response complexity according to success or difficulty with the previous perceptual activity (Erber 1976, 1977, 1980a; see Chapter 5).

Because the speech-perception process is hidden from view, most perceptual learning must be inferred. Even the child's *attention* to the task must be inferred from observable behavior. A child's head and body may be oriented to the task, although watching or listening is not taking place. Teaching experience is required to make correct inferences regarding a child's level of attention and readiness for perceptual learning.

VISUAL PERCEPTION

Attention to a speaker's facial and postural cues is important for perception of spoken language and development of natural social interaction (Argyle 1988). Visible cues often convey the speaker's intent and emotional state. Most children – either with normal hearing or impaired hearing – rely partly on their *vision* for language learning and for speech communication (Woodhouse et al., 2008).

Many hearing-impaired children use visual perception of the speaker's articulation to augment their imperfect auditory perception. The linguistic symbols received from lipreading are the visually observable positions and movements of the lips, teeth, tongue, and surrounding facial surfaces. Visual perception of a lip or tongue position alone, however, is usually not sufficient for accurate identification of a particular speech element. For example, a closure of the lips by itself has no linguistic value. It may even indicate an *absence* of communication (resting position). But if a child perceives lip closure in combination with a subsequent lip opening, then this sequence of movements becomes a visible indicator of a particular set of speech sounds in English (/p, b, m/).

Most speakers do not consciously create distinguishable mouth shapes as they talk, but instead produce acoustically correct *sounds*. Thus mouth shapes tend to be unconscious visible by-products of speech-sound production. Although, in general, hearing people are not aware of mouth shapes and movements (except when they try to lipread a speaker in a noisy place), most hearing-impaired children learn to use visible articulations as linguistic symbols (Alich 1967; De Filippo 1982).

Mouth shapes are less efficient language symbols than speech sounds or printed letters, however. There are several reasons.
- Some vowels cannot be distinguished visually because of similarities in lip spreading or rounding (e.g., /U/ and /u/).
- Some mouth shapes (e.g., upper teeth pressed to lower lip) are associated with more than one speech sound (e.g., /f/ and /v/).
- Some speech processes occur deep within the vocal tract and cannot be seen, such as the production of voice by a vibrating larynx (e.g., that distinguishes /z/

from /s/), or the production of nasality by lowering the soft palate (e.g., that distinguishes /n/ from /t, d/).

- "Co-articulation" influences the visibility of many speech units. Some mouth shapes that can be identified in isolation become indistinguishable when they occur in combination. For example, in the word *needles*, the phonetic elements /d/, /l/, and /z/ blend to form a single mouth shape (you might even suggest that all of the mouth shapes in this difficult word look the same).

There are about 40 speech sounds in spoken English. This number becomes 9 to 14 mouth shapes during conversational speech because many speech sounds look alike – either in isolation or in context (Jeffers & Barley 1971; Kricos & Lesner 1982).

INFORMATION AVAILABLE THROUGH LIPREADING

Despite these visual ambiguities, many hearing-impaired children learn spoken language by combining visual perception of oral and facial cues with auditory perception of acoustic cues they receive from their hearing aids or cochlear implants.

Vowel information

Although children differ in their ability to lipread vowels, most can distinguish between spread (front) and rounded (back) vowel categories. These two types of lip opening (e.g., as in the vowels /i/ and /u/) form very distinct mouth shapes. It is far more common for children to confuse vowels that are produced with similar lip openings (e.g., /i/ and /I/). Vowel identification has been shown to be relatively unaffected by viewing conditions such as distance, light level, or optical clarity (Erber 1971, 1974a, 1979a).

Consonant information

Most children can separate consonants into visibility groups based on *place* of articulation (e.g., labial, alveolar, velar). Visual recognition of consonants, however, is influenced by the context of adjacent vowels (Erber 1971). It is common for children to visually confuse consonants that look alike but differ by voicing or manner of articulation, such as /p, b, m/ (Erber 1972a).

Even inexperienced lipreaders can quickly learn to distinguish among the *places* of consonant articulation (Erber 1972a), and little specific practice seems necessary to reach this basic ability level (Walden et al., 1977). Accurate visual identification of other articulatory details in consonants, however, requires good viewing conditions (Erber 1971, 1974a).

Word information

Children generally identify longer words, such as spondees with two stressed syllables (*football*), more easily than shorter words with only one syllable (*cat*) (Erber 1971, 1974a). Two-syllable words with either iambic (*giraffe*) or trochaic (*father*) stress tend to be intermediate in intelligibility. It seems that the more (stressed) syllables a word contains, the more speech movements and visible contrasts are available for its identification. An important factor that contributes to the intelligibility of a word seems to be the uniqueness of its visible articulatory pattern – the extent to which the word "looks different" from other words in the language (e.g., *thumb*).

Sentence information

Children generally lipread short simple sentences more easily than long complex sentences (Clouser 1976). Complicated syntactic constructions, such as embedded clauses, passive verbs, negatives, multiple subjects or objects, question forms, or combinations of these make sentences more difficult to lipread (Schwartz & Black 1967). Hearing-impaired children seem to have the greatest success identifying sentences of the form subject-verb-object (prepositional phrase), probably because this is a basic construction with high utility.

A major limitation of lipreading is that co-articulation of speech sounds from adjacent words in a sentence often makes it difficult for a lipreader to specify word boundaries. This is especially true where reduced syllable stress affects the visible clarity of mouth movements. To comprehend a sentence through lipreading, a child must not only perceive speech rhythm and word emphasis, but also rely on context and knowledge of language for probable word sequences. This is why it is extremely difficult to learn spoken language through lipreading alone, and why cochlear implants provide such significant benefit for children with extreme hearing loss.

COMBINED AUDITORY-VISUAL PERCEPTION

The speech-perception skills of hearing-impaired children vary widely. Important auditory skills include the ability to hear prosody and intonation, voicing and nasality in consonants, and low-frequency formants in vowels. Some children with impaired hearing can distinguish vowel and consonant qualities nearly as well as children with normal hearing, and they can reliably identify familiar words. Others have difficulty distinguishing sound frequencies, and cannot hear details in vowels and consonants. Some are able to perceive only the intensity patterns of speech (Erber 1972a, 1972b, 1974b, 1979b; Zeiser & Erber, 1977; Boothroyd 1984).

Although some early intervention programs promote listening and discourage lipreading, most hearing-impaired children perceive speech better when they watch the speaker as they listen.

For many children, the ability to see the place of articulation of consonants and the mouth shapes of vowels complements the ability to distinguish low-frequency acoustic cues. Thus looking while listening can help a hearing-impaired child distinguish between the words *thin/fin, met/net,* or *teeth/tooth,* although the child may not be able to hear these differences by listening alone. The combination of both auditory and visual cues usually results in better perception of speech than can be achieved through either sense alone.

Even when visual information is added to auditory information, however, there are differences in speech perception between hearing-impaired children. A child who perceives only intensity patterns through an amplification system is likely to experience continuing difficulty in speech perception. Intensity patterns without significant frequency information do not supply enough acoustic detail to complement the visible place of articulation and mouth-shape information that can be obtained through lipreading. The perceptual information obtained from these two inputs may even overlap, as the intensity pattern of speech is related to changes in the size of the speaker's visible mouth opening (Grant & Seitz 2000).

A cochlear implant increases the auditory and auditory–visual communication potential of a child with a significant hearing loss, mainly because the device increases the child's awareness of important frequency details in speech (Geers, Brenner et al., 2003). When a cochlear implant is combined with an educational program that emphasizes speech and auditory skills, the child's opportunity for the development of spoken language is greatly increased (Moog 2002; Geers, Nicholas et al., 2003)

SUMMARY

A hearing-impaired child's ability to perceive speech, produce intelligible speech, and learn spoken language are all closely related to the child's ability to perceive the sound patterns and frequencies of speech. An appropriate personal listening system is a basic requirement. The child listens to acoustic models of spoken language, and learns to recognize when his/her imitations are correct. To perceive important features of speech, a typical hearing-impaired child listens to sound qualities and observes visible patterns. The parent and teacher must recognize the child's auditory abilities and limitations, and provide supportive strategies when necessary.

CHAPTER 3

The (re)habilitation process

The principal aim of an auditory approach to (re)habilitation is to help a hearing-impaired child learn to communicate through spoken language. Awareness and acquisition of spoken language depends on the child's ability to hear the speech of others as well as hear his/her own vocal output. A hearing impairment in a young child affects these processes, and may delay or modify both speech and language development.

The terms "acoupedics", "auditory training", "auditory-oral", and "auditory-verbal" have been used to describe a group of methods specifically intended to increase a hearing-impaired child's ability to perceive speech through listening (Beattie 2006). The aim is to enable the child to apply the sense of hearing in language acquisition and communication, regardless of the condition of the impaired auditory system. Usually, progress is achieved by applying suitable hearing aids or cochlear implants and through special teaching techniques (Pollack 1970; Erber 1982; Ling 1989; Nevins & Chute 1996; Moog 2002; Schery & Peters 2003). The therapy process may include identifying auditory abilities, reducing visible cues for speech, presenting a variety of listening tasks, and applying strategies to help the child acquire auditory communication skills. This chapter supplies a rationale for these techniques.

Figure 3.1 summarizes the main components of an auditory approach to communication development. Although the process is shown as a series of steps, assessment and therapy are often combined, and there is much overlap between the various components.

ASSESS THE CHILD'S HEARING

Most hearing-test batteries for children include procedures summarised in figure 3.1 and discussed below.

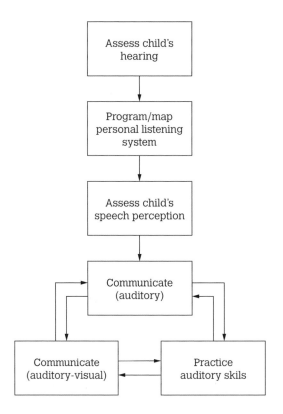

Figure 3.1 **Flow chart of auditory assessment, communication, and practice**

Outer-ear examination

The clinician uses an otoscope (illuminated magnifier) to look for cerumen (ear wax) that can block the ear canal, and also to check for obvious outer- or middle-ear problems (e.g., skin irritation, perforated eardrum, or otitis media). If cerumen or signs of an ear disorder are present, the child should be referred to a physician. Cerumen should always be removed by a qualified person, such as a doctor or nurse.

Tympanometry

Middle-ear disease can impede transmission of sound to the inner ear and produce a conductive hearing loss. Tympanometry is a technique used to test the condition of the middle ear and mobility of the eardrum (Northern & Downs 2002). A rubber seal is placed in the child's ear canal and sound is introduced through a small tube. Air pressure is slowly changed in the ear canal, and the amount of sound reflected from the eardrum is measured. This method can detect middle-ear conditions related to eardrum stiffness or abnormal pressure, such as fluid in the middle ear, or a blocked eustacian tube. If a middle-ear condition is found, the child is referred to a doctor for treatment.

Audiometry

Audiometry is a method for describing hearing in terms of the softest tones the child can detect at different sound frequencies (Northern & Downs 2002). Newborns are assessed by placing electrodes on the child's head, and measuring the brain's electrical output to sound from small earphones. Infants are tested with *visual reinforcement audiometry*, in which they respond to sounds from a loudspeaker by turning the head to view a moving toy. Pre-school children can be evaluated through *play audiometry* where the child manipulates an object (e.g., puts a toy in a box) when a test sound is detected. School-age children can listen through earphones and respond by raising a hand or finger.

The result is a graph (audiogram) of the child's sensitivity to tones at different frequencies, relative to normal sensitivity (0 dB HL). The audiogram usually is superimposed on a shaded area that depicts the range of sound frequencies and intensities that occur in conversational speech (the speech area) (see figure 3.2). The complete diagram describes in general the frequencies and intensities of speech the child can probably detect, and thus indicates the need for a personal listening system (e.g., hearing aids, cochlear implants). Repeated testing is used to monitor changes in the child's hearing sensitivity over time.

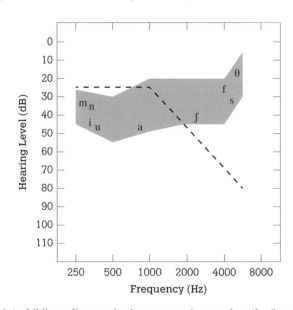

Figure 3.2 **A child's audiogram is shown superimposed on the "speech area"**

Although the child listens to pure tones and not speech, the procedure is useful for identifying factors that can affect the child's development of speech-communication skills such as audibility of low and/or high frequency sounds. Audiologists tend to rely on pure-tone audiometry for determining the most appropriate personal listening system for each child, for programming/mapping the device, and making decisions regarding educational planning.

PROGRAM/MAP PERSONAL LISTENING SYSTEM

For most children with impaired hearing, there is little opportunity for detecting and interpreting the sounds of speech unless a personal listening system (typically hearing aids or cochlear implants) is used to increase the audibility of these sounds. An important step in any auditory communication program is the selection, programming, and functional evaluation of the child's personal listening system.

Hearing aids

A hearing aid is a miniature amplification system that contains a small microphone, amplifier, earphone, and battery. Most children use the behind-the-ear (BTE) type, where sound output is delivered to the ear canal through a small plastic tube held in place by an earmold.

Hearing aid selection for a young hearing-impaired child can be a challenge, because the child often lacks the vocabulary or language required to describe the auditory sensations. The child may not be able to tell the audiologist when speech is audible, which hearing aid adjustments produce the greatest speech clarity, or when over-amplification produces distortion or discomfort. Despite these obstacles, an audiologist is able to select and program hearing aids for a young child based on:

- recommendations provided by the manufacturer
- evidence-based formulae that prescribe optimal sound output for the child's hearing loss
- measurement of sound levels produced by the aids in the child's ear canals
- clinical experience with other children who use hearing aids
- parents' descriptions of the child's auditory behavior.

For very young children, the amount of amplification at each frequency is usually calculated to increase the level of sound for best perception and listening comfort (Dillon 2001; Seewald et al., 2005). For older children who have developed auditory speech-perception abilities, the audiologist can use speech sounds, words, and sentences to verify previous decisions regarding hearing aid programming.

Cochlear implants

Children with profound hearing impairments may derive minimal benefit from hearing aids. Despite sound amplification, they may be unable to distinguish sound frequencies and may perceive only rhythmic intensity patterns in speech. These children are candidates for cochlear implants if they meet other criteria, including:

- hearing loss detected early
- normal inner ear anatomy
- parental desire for speech communication
- realistic expectations
- strong family support
- availability of educational support services.

A cochlear implant is a complex electronic device used to restore auditory sensation and perception to a child with a significant hearing loss. An array of tiny electrodes is surgically placed within the child's cochlea (inner ear). Sound is detected by a head-worn microphone and encoded as electrical pulses by a small digital signal processor. These electrical pulses are presented to the electrodes in the child's inner ear and stimulate the auditory nerve directly.

The implant's sound processor must be adjusted ("mapped") to suit the individual child. Mapping an implant involves setting each electrode's stimulation levels for soft and comfortably loud speech – to permit perception of a wide range of sounds in daily life. The child's pure-tone thresholds are obtained while listening through the implant system. Comfortable listening levels are judged by the child, or estimated by the audiologist according to a prescribed formula. The ability to detect and/or discriminate a variety of speech sounds also may be evaluated. Periodic adjustments may be required to optimize listening levels. After implantation and listening experience, most children are able to perceive a greater range of sound qualities than before, and they acquire a much greater potential for development of auditory communication skills (Boothroyd & Boothroyd-Turner 2002; Moog 2002; Geers, Nicholas et al., 2003; Geers et al., 2011).

Post-fitting/post-implantation

Following hearing aid fitting or cochlear implant surgery, careful observation of the child's auditory responses and communication behavior is vital. The child's parents and therapist/teacher observe the child at home and in the clinic/(pre-) school as the child uses the amplification system programmed to initial settings. In addition to these subjective judgments, tests are also performed to establish the child's responsiveness to speech. Evaluation of a child's personal listening system is an ongoing process that continues for many years.

Following hearing aid fitting or cochlear implantation, the child and his/her parents must learn routine procedures to maintain proper functioning of the apparatus. These include avoiding physical damage, keeping components dry and in good condition, regular testing and replacing (or recharging) batteries, and cleaning cerumen from earmolds (Chute & Nevins 2002; Hedley-Williams et al., 2003). Daily checks are recommended. To simplify this process, the child can be taught vocabulary and language associated with routine maintenance, such as *hear, sound, switch, cord, earmold, battery, processor.*

Use of a personal listening system

Audiologists consider many factors when they recommend hearing aids or cochlear implants.

Binaural vs monaural listening

Audiologists typically recommend that personal listening systems be fitted to both ears. Binaural delivery of sound usually provides greater benefit than delivery of sound to a single ear alone because (Dillon 2001):

- more acoustic information is available
- directional hearing permits location of a sound source
- speech is more apparent in background noise.

Speech quality

Digital programmable listening devices offer the flexibility to match the amount of amplified sound to each child's hearing loss, suppress background noise, and control feedback squeal. Wireless/FM amplification systems often are used to assist children in kindergartens or classrooms. A microphone can be placed near the speaker's mouth, and a high-quality speech signal can be delivered to the child's ears, even in the presence of background noise.

Listening environment

The content and quality of sound that enters the child's listening system are very important. To be effective, not only must the device be in good working condition, but the surrounding environment must be reasonably quiet, and the speaker must be relatively close to the child. The speaker's message must also be timely, meaningful, and clearly articulated.

Underuse or rejection

Some children underuse or even reject their hearing aids/cochlear implants. Some reasons include late fitting of the listening system, limited communication benefit, reported unpleasant sensation of sound, and/or embarrassment about appearing different (Watson & Gregory 2005; Archbold et al., 2009).

ASSESSING AND FACILITATING SPEECH PERCEPTION

Basic hearing test results provide an estimate of a child's potential for perceiving the sound qualities of speech. Parents and therapists use this information to structure a program for assessing and facilitating the child's speech-perception skills.

Infants

In a typical early intervention program, parents learn how to communicate with their children and help them develop listening skills, spoken language, self-monitoring, and social interaction (Clezy 1984; Simmons-Martin & Rossi 1990; Simser 1999; Calderon 2000; Harrigan & Nikolopoulos 2002). Detailed tests of speech perception in infants are not usually conducted in the hearing clinic. Instead, a therapist shows parents how to informally monitor their child's development as a listener and communicator. "Diagnostic teaching" procedures are used to assess progress.

Older children

A wide range of standard tests are available to evaluate speech perception in older children: detection of speech sounds; identification of monosyllabic words; identification of key words in sentences. The results indicate how well the child responds to spoken materials, and the findings can be compared with results obtained from other children. Repeated testing is used to monitor the child's progress over time. Chapter 4 covers this topic in greater detail.

It is important to note that a child's poor performance on a speech perception test may sometimes be due to factors such as:

- misunderstanding the test instructions
- insufficient attention to the task
- insufficient vocabulary or language
- listening through a system that is not working properly
- insufficient listening experience.

Careful observation and repeated testing with different speech materials are required for confident conclusions and recommendations. After a basic description of the child's hearing is obtained, listening activities can be selected to extend the range of speech perception skills. See Chapters 5 and 6 for more detail.

AUDITORY AND AUDITORY-VISUAL COMMUNICATION

Natural face-to-face (auditory-visual) communication and specific listening (auditory only) practice can usually be combined without disrupting spoken interaction between the child and adult. When a parent or therapist is helping a young child develop listening skills, the adult can either sit beside the child, or obscure the mouth to minimize visual cues and direct the child's attention to the *sounds* of speech. An experienced adult can easily shift between auditory-visual and auditory-only communication, simply by obscuring the mouth during selected parts of an utterance.

Regardless of the amount of hearing loss, listening system, or method of instruction, most hearing-impaired children perceive speech with greater accuracy when they receive both auditory and visual input simultaneously, rather than just auditory or visual cues alone (Erber 1975; Lachs et al., 2001; Bergeson et al., 2004). Some children gain sufficient information from listening alone, if their hearing is adequate and the conditions are optimal, but most prefer to lipread as they listen. Teachers in regular schools are generally advised to make sure that they are both audible and visible whenever they speak. This is especially important when presenting material that contains new language, new vocabulary, or important details.

Auditory skills matrix

A variety of communication options are available to an adult while interacting with a hearing-impaired child. The auditory skills matrix (see figure 3.3) summarizes types of speech *stimulus* (e.g., spoken words or sentences) that a hearing-impaired child might receive in conversation with family, friends, teachers, or therapists. The diagram also shows the types of *response* (e.g., identification, comprehension) that might be expected in each case. This stimulus-response matrix will be used to guide our general approach to assessment and auditory skills practice (Erber 1976, 1980a, 1982; Erber & Hirsh 1978).

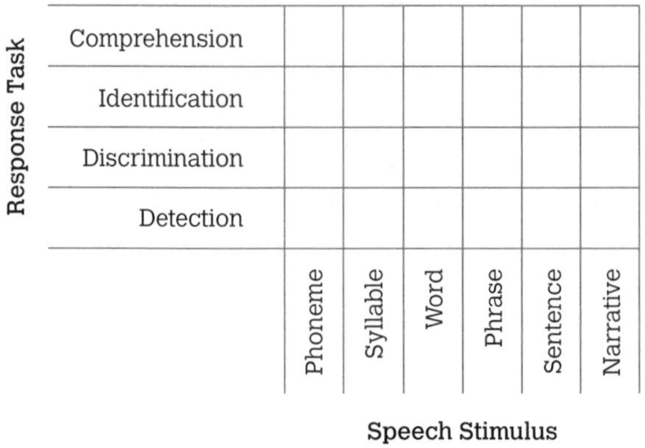

Response Task		Phoneme	Syllable	Word	Phrase	Sentence	Narrative
	Comprehension						
	Identification						
	Discrimination						
	Detection						

Speech Stimulus

Figure 3.3 **Auditory skills matrix illustrating the range of speech stimulus items and response tasks**

As we examine this diagram from left to right, we see that the units of speech become longer and linguistically more complex. As we progress from bottom to top, we observe that response tasks increase in difficulty. A child's ability to respond at each level can be viewed as a component of the next level of listening. For example, similar speech sounds (e.g., the consonants θ, ʃ, and tʃ) must be detected before they can be discriminated from one another. Similar words (e.g., *with, wish, witch*) must be heard and discriminated as different from one another before they can be reliably named and identified.

Each box in the diagram represents the combination of a particular type of spoken speech stimulus and a specific behavioral response. For example, a child might be requested to tell whether the two phrases *under the books* and *into the bush* sound the same or whether they are different, which is a discrimination task. The child might be asked to repeat the sentence "These shoes are too big!", which is an identification task. Nearly all communication tasks can be analyzed and located in the matrix in this way. Auditory tests and listening activities can be created to fit into any stimulus-response box shown in figure 3.3.

Ideally, to completely evaluate a hearing-impaired child's auditory speech-perception skills, a specific test would be administered for each stimulus-response combination depicted in this diagram. That is, to describe a child's auditory status in detail, we should obtain complete descriptive and diagnostic information for every box in the matrix. After we identify which auditory stimulus-response tasks seem relatively easy for the child, we can direct listening practice primarily to those tasks on which the child demonstrates greater difficulty.

To obtain a complete description of a child's speech-perception abilities, however, an audiologist would need to present at least 24 separate tests (six types of stimulus and four levels of response) – each administered under several listening conditions.

Four levels of response to an acoustic speech stimulus:
- Detection – can you hear this?
- Discrimination – does this sound different from that?
- Identification – what did you hear?
- Comprehension – what does it mean?

This amount of measurement is impractical, especially for young children, so we tend to substitute careful observation (diagnostic teaching) for objective testing in most cases. This approach is valid and reliable when performed by experienced teachers or therapists. Some specific tests may also be needed to obtain a quick estimate of the child's current speech perception ability (see Chapter 4).

Continuum of stimulus materials

The items that you can use to evaluate and facilitate a child's auditory speech perception range from very simple to very complex. At one end of the continuum are individual speech sounds, syllables, and words, all of which are widely used by audiologists during hearing assessment. These brief units of speech are frequently used because:
- many test items can be presented within a short time
- responses can easily be scored "right" or "wrong"
- items can be presented in a multiple-choice ("closed set") format
- a child's perceptual errors may be explained on the basis of "speech feature" analysis.

The main objection to the use of such simple speech materials is that they do not represent the content of most daily conversation, although a child's responses to simple items may be related to higher levels of auditory communication.

At the other end of the speech continuum are phrases, sentences, and narrative, all of which are desirable as test materials because they represent the content of daily conversation. The main difficulty with using complex test items like this concerns the scoring of responses to large language units (such as sentences). Some teachers and therapists feel that a child should be rewarded for identifying the main idea of a spoken message, although it is more reliable to score responses to complete sentences or designated key words as "right" or "wrong".

Comprehension of longer units of spoken language (such as phrases, sentences, or narrative) involves both perception of sound *and* knowledge of language. Sentences are constructed according to rules of syntax (word order) and semantics (meaning), and they are often redundant and predictable. A child may appear to comprehend an entire sentence, although the child has heard and identified only a fragment. Most sentences that occur in the context of a conversation are related in some way. For all these reasons, careful interpretation of test results is necessary.

Continuum of response tasks

Detection tasks

Detection is the act of determining whether sound is present or absent. The child's response may take the form of turning the head or eyes toward the sound to obtain more information, or an audiologist may specifically ask the child to perform a particular observable task (place a toy in a box, raise a hand or finger) whenever sound is detected. Awareness of sound in daily life helps maintain contact with the surrounding acoustic environment, and alerts the child that something is happening. Awareness of sound also is important for learning the relationships between people or objects and the sounds they produce.

Audiologists use detection responses, not only to obtain a child's pure-tone thresholds, but also to establish minimal requirements for sound amplification through a personal listening system. Teachers and therapists also employ detection tasks to determine which speech sounds are audible to a hearing-impaired child under particular acoustic conditions (e.g., in locations that are quiet or noisy, or at different distances). For example, the adult may ask the child, "Can you hear this sound ... /a/, /f/, /m/, ...?" When a child listens through a personal listening system, the stronger speech sounds may be audible, but the weaker sounds may reach the child's level of awareness only at a near distance.

Discrimination tasks

Discrimination is the ability to hear differences (and similarities) in intensity, duration, and quality between speech sounds. Even if the child can detect most speech sounds, hearing is of little value for communication unless sounds can be distinguished from one another.

Discrimination of sounds and subjective grouping of sounds into categories are complementary abilities. To describe several sounds as the "same", a child must place them into a common perceptual category compared to other sounds judged to be "different". Initially all sounds may seem similar to a young child with little or no listening experience, although the sounds can be distinguished from silence. Later, the child learns that sounds differ in many ways: loud/soft, long/short, high pitch/low pitch, and so forth.

The concepts of "same" and "different" can be relative, depending on the context in which the spoken items are presented. The words *duck* and duck spoken by two different people may be described as the "same" in one context ("which is different? *duck*, duck, *apple*") but probably would be described as "different" under other test conditions ("which is different?: *duck*, duck, *duck*").

Most teachers and therapists apply discrimination tasks *remedially*, that is, to learn more about a child's perceptual difficulty when the child makes an error on an auditory identification task. For example, the topic may be gardening. The teacher says, "We planted an apple *seed*. What did we plant?" The child responds "*fruit*". The teacher may present the word that she spoke and the child's incorrect response together, and ask: "Do these words sound the same or different?: *seed* ..... *fruit*." The purpose is to find out whether the child is unable to hear the difference between the confused words, or does not know that the two sound patterns represent different concepts and should be labeled differently.

Identification tasks

Identification responses, commonly obtained in clinical hearing assessments, are labels (names) for what the child has heard. The child may indicate identification of a spoken item by repeating, pointing to a toy/picture, or writing the word or sentence that was perceived. For example, a teacher might ask a hearing-impaired child to "Show me the *bear*!" or to repeat an entire sentence: "The children played football in the park". These types of identification response require the child to recall and name the item that was spoken.

An identification response may be *segmental*, where the child describes the spoken item exactly (points to a picture of a cup after hearing the spoken word "cup"). Or, the identification response may be *suprasegmental*, where the child describes the acoustic pattern without actually naming the spoken word (points to a symbolic representation of a single syllable after hearing the spoken word "cup") (Chute & Nevins 2002). Other suprasegmental identification tasks include: indicating the location of acoustic stress in a word or sentence; labeling a sentence as "short" or "long"; or pointing out the location of a brief pause in a sentence. These are examples of auditory abilities that are relevant to extraction of meaning in sentences.

Auditory identification of spoken language units is related to the child's growing awareness that people (*girl*), things (*food*), and activities (*eat*) have names, and that each name can be represented as an acoustic pattern. In addition, the child learns that the sounds people and objects produce also have names (*shout, buzz, roar*), and that these words also are important for communication through speech.

In general, a teacher would use an identification task to determine how a spoken stimulus was perceived by a hearing-impaired child. For example, if the child fails to answer a question or follow an instruction correctly, you may ask the child to *repeat* the question or instruction. The response may indicate whether the problem lies in understanding your intended meaning or in identifying (or remembering) what you said. You can create identification tests to diagnose specific listening difficulties. For example, you can use sentences that differ in length, redundancy, or syntactic complexity to discover how particular language patterns and structures influence the child's ability to identify (and thus respond to) your requests (Kalikow et al., 1977).

Comprehension tasks

Comprehension of speech requires that the child understand the meaning of a spoken message, usually by reference to knowledge of language and previous experience. A child with auditory comprehension skills can acquire new concepts through hearing and can think, feel, and act appropriately. To verify that auditory comprehension has occurred, a comprehension response must differ in content from an identification response. That is, the child cannot simply repeat what you said. Instead, the child must demonstrate understanding with a response that differs from what you said, but is closely associated in some way. For example, if you ask Daniel, "What is your name?", and he repeats, "What is your name?", he has demonstrated only *identification* of what you said. In contrast, if the child responds with "Daniel!", then he has demonstrated *comprehension* of your question.

Other examples of comprehension tasks include complying with requests, such as, "Please give some of your popcorn to Liz!", or "Draw a picture of a house with lots of windows!" A word-comprehension task might require the child to say the opposite of *hot, tall, happy*, and so forth. Often, a teacher will informally promote a child's auditory comprehension by giving instructions or asking questions with the mouth obscured.

Comprehension is a prerequisite for auditory-only communication, such as:
- listening to a teacher while writing notes
- listening to a description while watching a demonstration
- listening to voice-over narration on television
- participating in conversation over the telephone.

FACTORS THAT CAN AFFECT A CHILD'S RESPONSE TO SPEECH

Many factors can affect the ease with which a child responds to a particular speech stimulus. These include:
- clarity – e.g., speaker's voice pitch, articulatory precision, intensity, rate, syllable stress, pauses
- speech patterns – e.g., prosody, intonation, syllabic structure
- number of units in the utterance – e.g., syllables, words, phrases, clauses, sentences
- complexity of the utterance – i.e., simple versus complex

- surrounding environment – e.g., quiet, noisy, distracting
- distance between the speaker and the child.

AUDITORY GOALS

Auditory goals change as a child grows. Parents are usually an infant's main communication partners, and the home is the main learning environment. Parents are encouraged to speak to the child during all daily activities. Environmental sounds and speech are important parts of the young child's life experience and auditory development.

At first, sound awareness is a primary concern. Then the child begins to associate sound patterns with particular play activities (e.g., "Ring around the rosie ..."). The child is encouraged to develop auditory memory for increasingly longer sound sequences. The sounds of speech become an important part of early social interaction and later conversational exchanges.

A teacher or therapist may be an older child's main source of auditory learning, although of course there is much daily interaction with parents, siblings, and friends. Auditory communication occurs in a variety of environments both within and outside the home. Auditory communication becomes a medium for social contact and a source of information. Listening is required for learning at school. Acquisition of vocabulary and complex language is a continuing process. Intelligible speech is necessary for fluent interaction with others, and so auditory self-monitoring becomes very important.

AUDITORY DEVELOPMENT STRATEGIES

Both research and experience indicate that in order to maximize the intelligibility of spoken messages, a parent or teacher should routinely use clear speech and language, including precise articulation, slow syllable rate, common words, and short, simple declarative sentences (Uchanski 2005). Parents and teachers, however, must do more than present easily understood sentences. To ensure vocabulary/language learning and cognitive development, a hearing-impaired child's auditory speech-perception abilities must be *challenged*. This is done by presenting more complex language structures that the child may not immediately understand through listening alone.

Most adults tend to apply one of two general approaches to a hearing-impaired child's auditory communication and learning. Some adults speak ordinary sentences with little conscious management of the vocabulary or syntax. If the child does not understand, they repeat, clarify, or simplify the utterance according to the child's specific needs (Erber & Greer 1973; Erber 1996; Nevins & Chute 1996). This strategy typically involves the use of "natural language" and the remediation of any observed difficulties. An alternative approach involves presenting vocabulary and sentence structures that are known to be within the communication capabilities of the child. When the child demonstrates understanding, the adult supplies a more complex sentence or a related question. This is an "extension" approach based on awareness of the child's present level of competence and the conscious introduction of increasingly complex language (Kenworthy 1986; Pianta & Stuhlman 2004; DesJardin & Eisenberg 2007).

Adaptive communication

Many parents, therapists, and teachers *combine* the extension and remediation methods in what may be called "adaptive communication" (Erber 1977). To use this method, an adult considers each communication exchange with a child as an informal auditory "test" with particular levels of stimulus and response. This type of simple evaluation becomes a part of daily interaction. The child's responses indicate whether the child is able to function adequately at the level of stimulus-response difficulty that the adult has chosen. The stimulus-response matrix described earlier (see figure 3.3) can be used as a framework to implement this approach. Within this framework, how you choose each auditory communication task will vary according to whether your previous choices produced positive outcomes. That is, what you say and how you say it will depend on the child's success with what you said before.

If the hearing-impaired child seems to perceive your auditory communication with no difficulty at a particular level of vocabulary and sentence complexity, then you will either maintain communication at that level, or you may *adapt* by introducing new vocabulary or more complex language. If, however, the child demonstrates difficulty in responding appropriately to what you have said, first you will need to determine what the problem is. For example:
- the child may not have been paying attention
- you may have spoken without clarity
- you may have presented unfamiliar vocabulary or complex sentence structure
- the child may have misinterpreted the situational context
- you may have required a response beyond the child's capabilities.

Then you will need to adapt. For example, you may:
- gain the child's attention
- speak more clearly
- substitute more familiar vocabulary and/or language
- specify/clarify the situational context
- request a lower-level response (or provide visible cues).

This approach is summarized in figure 3.4. In general, the more difficult listening activities are located in the upper right area of this diagram. Easier auditory tasks appear in the lower left area. The aim is to help the hearing-impaired child maximize hearing, ultimately to perform the tasks in the upper right area of the matrix, which are part of daily conversation (e.g., comprehension of sentences and narrative).

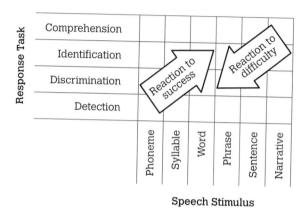

Figure 3.4 **Auditory skills matrix illustrating the dynamic nature of "adaptive communication". Each listening activity is selected according to the child's success with previous tasks**

Initially, the adult will observe the child's responses to auditory communication tasks in different situations. The boundary between "easy" and "difficult" listening for a particular child will lie somewhere between the upper right and lower left corners. Most listening activities will take place in this boundary region. The adult will present a listening task at a particular level of difficulty, observe the child's response, and then choose the next listening task based on the child's success or difficulty.

For example, during an auditory word-identification game, you may say a word (e.g., "dog"), and ask the child to listen and point to an appropriate picture. If the child shows no difficulty with this listening task, you may try increasing the length or complexity of what you say (e.g., a sentence containing the key word: "The brown *dog* is playing with the boys"), and continue to ask the child to point to (identify) an appropriate picture. Alternatively, you may ask questions about each picture (e.g., "What color is *that* dog?"), and elicit spoken comprehension responses.

If, however, the child fails to comprehend a spoken request, such as "Put your toys in the box!", you may simplify by presenting only the phrase "in the box". Alternatively, the child's response may be simplified by requiring only *identification* of your request: "Put your toys in the box .... What did I say?" At another time, the child may respond "in my bedroom!" to your question, "When do you watch TV?" implying that *when* was identified as *where*. In this case, you can simplify the response from comprehension to discrimination by pairing the two confused words and asking: "Do these words sound the same? when ... where". These are examples of an adaptive approach to auditory communication.

An adaptive approach to auditory communication requires you to:

- continuously evaluate the child's auditory speech-perception abilities
- relate each communication activity to the child's auditory skills
- identify the stimulus-response elements of each spoken interchange (see figure 3.3)
- know how to present a variety of developmental/remedial listening activities, as described in later chapters
- be able to quickly modify clarity, complexity, and content as you communicate with the child.

Further information on the adaptive communication approach is contained in Chapter 5.

SUMMARY

A general sequence for auditory skills development includes:

- audiometric evaluation
- selecting/programming/mapping the child's personal listening system
- assessing the child's auditory speech-perception skills
- auditory and auditory-visual communication according to the child's abilities and needs
- informal assessment and adaptation during regular communication.

CHAPTER 4

Adaptive hearing assessment

During auditory testing, a hearing-impaired child may be unable to detect particular speech sounds (e.g., /f, s, θ/) or may be unable to identify some common words (e.g., *ball, bird, cat, soap, teeth, tongue, cake*). The child may obtain a low score, for example, 20 or 30 per cent words correct. The child's parents and family members may be surprised by results like these, and want advice. It is likely that they would want to know how to communicate effectively with the child in spite of the child's auditory errors.

In this chapter, we will describe a simple method for assessing speech perception that informs adults and guides them as communication partners. This method, called Adaptive Hearing Assessment (AHA!), is not suggested as an alternative to current diagnostic methods, but is proposed as a supplementary procedure. The child's frequent communication partners (parents, therapists, teachers) can easily apply the results as they seek to develop the child's listening and spoken language skills.

STANDARD SPEECH PERCEPTION TESTS

Audiologists and therapists generally conduct speech perception tests with a child and examine the test results before commencing an auditory learning program. They do this to better understand the child's strengths and weaknesses and to establish a baseline level of performance against which to measure future progress. Many test formats and test materials are available to describe a child's speech perception abilities. Some examples include:

- detection of speech sounds: 5-sound and 6-sound test (Ling & Ling 1978; Ling 2003)
- same-different discrimination of speech sounds: THRIFT (Boothroyd, Springer et al., 1988)
- speech-feature perception tests (Merklein 1981; Boothroyd 1984; Maltby 2000)

- identification of words in a closed set: WIPI (Ross & Lerman 1979); NU-CHIPS (Elliott & Katz 1980)
- identification of words in an open set: PBK (Haskins 1949); AB lists (Boothroyd 1968, 1984)
- identification of words in a sentence context: BKB sentences (Bench et al., 1979)
- multi-level tests: LIP (Nikolopoulos et al., 2000); ESP (Moog & Geers 1990); EARS (Allum et al., 2000).

Careful test selection is important to ensure that testing is appropriate to the child. Most speech perception tests are designed for children in a specific age range, or with particular language abilities. Each type of speech perception test is also intended for a specific purpose. For example, individual speech sounds are presented to verify that the child can detect (and perhaps recognize) a wide range of acoustic details. Words are presented to determine whether the child can hear and identify the phonetic composition of basic vocabulary items. Sentences are used as stimulus material to determine whether the child can identify and understand grammatical sequences of related words.

Speech perception tests are presented either in a "closed-set" or "open-set" format. In a closed-set format, a small group of test items (and/or related pictures) is shown to the child, the examiner speaks one of the items, and the child must select from the set of alternatives. In an open-set format, no group of alternative choices is provided, and the child must rely on acoustic cues alone to produce a response. In general, open-set auditory tests are more difficult than closed-set tests and yield lower scores.

Before testing begins, it is usually necessary to demonstrate the test procedure to the child, for example, when to listen and how to respond. In a typical test sequence, the examiner first presents an acoustic stimulus (e.g., a speech sound, word, or sentence) and the child then responds as required (e.g., points to a picture, or repeats the stimulus) (see figure 4.1). The examiner judges and records whether the child's response was correct or incorrect.

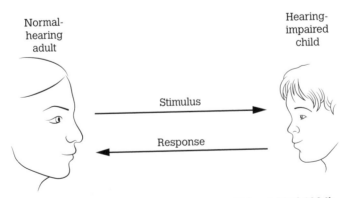

Figure 4.1 **Typical auditory test sequence (Erber & Lind 1994)**

Most speech perception tests yield numerical data that can be used to describe a child's current auditory status and to quantify changes in the child's listening skills over time. Test results provide evidence to support the choice of a particular listening system, programming/mapping strategy, or instructional method. Most tests yield per cent-correct scores that can be used to compare the effects of different listening systems and acoustic conditions.

In order to ensure that the test results reflect changes in the child's auditory performance and not variations in the spoken stimulus items, the test conditions and method of test presentation are usually prescribed and sound levels are carefully monitored. Each test item is delivered through headphones or a loudspeaker, the child's responses are obtained, and scores are assigned to the results. In many cases, an audio recording of the stimulus materials (e.g., a list of test words) is used to ensure stability of the acoustic patterns. The emphasis is on accuracy of measurement. To describe a child's speech perception skills in even greater detail, test items may be presented at different sound levels, in quiet/background noise, or with/without visible cues (Madell 1996; Bones & Diggory 1999).

The results of speech perception testing, however, may be of little direct value to the child's parents and teachers without interpretation. The child's responses are examined by the audiologist, who explains the child's auditory errors. For example:

- race > ray : the child could not detect the speech sound /s/
- comb > cone : the child misperceived the speech sound /m/
- fish > milk : the child perceived nonsense (ishk?) and responded with a familiar word.

CONVERSATIONAL INTERACTION

As discussed before, standard speech perception testing follows a carefully prescribed sequence: the examiner presents an acoustic stimulus, and the child responds by repeating the item or pointing to a corresponding picture (see figure 4.1). In real life, however, conversational exchange between a hearing-impaired child and an adult rarely follows such a simple stimulus > response sequence. Instead, the child may initiate the interaction with a statement, question, request, or a type of non-verbal behavior (e.g., the child pulls the adult's arm). When the adult recognizes that the child wants something, the adult speaks. The child may then indicate a lack of understanding through an inappropriate response, a confused facial expression, or a spoken request for help. Usually the adult repeats and/or clarifies to help the child understand. The child may require several types of clarification or communicative assistance before responding as desired to the adult's spoken "stimulus". This sequence is summarized in figure 4.2.

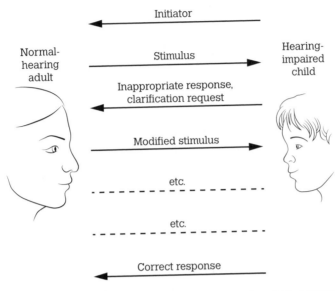

Figure 4.2 **Typical conversational sequence (Erber & Lind 1994)**

GASP!

The Glendonald Auditory Screening Procedure (GASP!) (Erber 1982) is a testing process that describes a child's listening skills, not only in terms of how many items are perceived correctly, but also in terms of the *adaptive strategies* applied by the examiner to help the child succeed as a listener. It is a simple assessment procedure that can be used to quickly estimate which auditory tasks can and cannot be performed easily, and which support strategies may be useful to help the child communicate. These results enable the adult to provide listening practice with tasks that are near the child's present auditory capabilities.

The auditory skills matrix shown in figure 3.3 illustrates six types of speech stimulus and four types of response that occur during conversation. The GASP! includes auditory tests based on three stimulus-response locations in the matrix (see figure 4.3):

1 speech-sound detection
2 word identification
3 sentence comprehension.

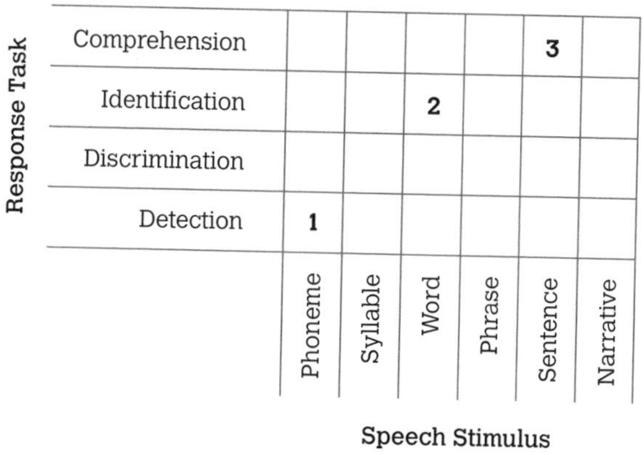

	Phoneme	Syllable	Word	Phrase	Sentence	Narrative
Comprehension					3	
Identification			2			
Discrimination						
Detection	1					

Response Task (vertical axis) — Speech Stimulus (horizontal axis)

Figure 4.3 **Auditory skills matrix. Locations of three types of auditory test are shown (adapted from Erber 1982)**

Three types of stimulus (speech sounds, words, sentences) and three types of response (detection, identification, comprehension) are represented by this choice.

It is recommended that a parent, therapist, or teacher present the GASP! tests because the child usually communicates with that person. For similar reasons, this live-voice assessment procedure should be administered through the personal listening system that the child normally uses (hearing aids, cochlear implants, wireless FM device).

Adaptive assessment is not a new concept. Many previous auditory tests and (re)-habilitation procedures have incorporated an adaptive component. For example:
- pure-tone threshold testing (Bekesy 1947; Northern & Downs 2002)
- word-identification testing (Bode & Carhart 1974; Mackie & Dermody 1986)
- sentence-identification testing (Erber 1992a)
- teachers' communication strategies (Erber & Greer 1973)
- tracking procedure (De Filippo & Scott 1978; Owens & Telleen 1981; Owens & Raggio 1987; Gnosspelius & Spens 1992)
- communication therapy (Erber 1984, 1988, 1996, 2002).

GASP! SUBTEST 1: AUDITORY DETECTION OF SPEECH SOUNDS

The first part of the GASP! is a speech-sound (*phoneme*) detection test. It evaluates the child's ability to detect speech sounds by listening alone. This subtest is related to aspects of verbotonal audiometry (Guberina 1964) and to the Ling 6-sound Test (see Ling 2003).

We use a speech-detection test for several reasons:
- to verify that the child's amplification system is working properly
- to determine if most speech sounds are audible
- to establish whether the adult's speech level is adequate for auditory communication at a near distance
- to indicate whether a therapist can confidently use acoustic modeling to modify the child's speech. (This topic is covered in more detail in Chapter 7.)

Standard test procedure

Placement. Sit at a table, opposite the child. Attach an outline picture of two small hands to the table in front of the child (see figure 4.4). This picture indicates where the hands should be placed when the child is not pointing to a response choice. Most young children will naturally place their hands within the outlines.

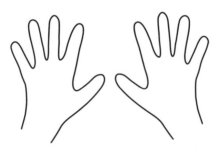

Figure 4.4 **Outline of hands used during testing (adapted from Erber 1982)**

YES/NO responses. Next, place two pictures of cartoon faces with open mouths before the child (see figure 4.5). These outlines are similar, but one face is shown with lines radiating from the mouth to indicate the production of sound; the other is shown with no lines, to indicate silence. The picture containing the lines is labeled YES. The picture without lines is labeled NO.

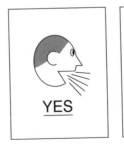
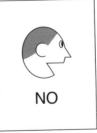

YES   NO

Figure 4.5 **Yes/No face pictures used during testing (adapted from Erber 1982)**

Stimulus items. Create a list of vowels (no diphthongs) and continuant consonants (no stop-plosives or affricates) as shown in figure 4.7. It is important to ensure that the sounds sampled cover a wide range of frequencies. Be sure to include a sample word with each vowel as a guide to its pronunciation. Also, divide the consonants into groups by manner of articulation, that is, nasal, lateral, voiced fricative, unvoiced fricative, etc. The list should also contain a blank space to indicate that occasionally you will produce a test item with appropriate articulation but produce *no* sound.

Create two rows of boxes to accompany the list of speech sounds and label these YES and NO. The child's responses should be recorded in these boxes, using the *same* mark (•) to indicate either a YES or NO response. Neither you, nor the child, should consider a NO response as "bad" or "incorrect" behavior. A NO response merely indicates that the child cannot detect a particular speech sound produced in isolation under test conditions.

Listening conditions. Make a written note of the listening system used by the child during the test: for example, hearing aids, cochlear implants, wireless FM device. Also make a note describing the amount of noise and/or other distractions in the test environment. For best test results, the conditions should be optimal.

Preliminary instructions. Before you assess speech-sound detection, you will need to teach the child what to do. First, say to the child: "I want you to listen (point to your ear). If you hear something (nod your head *yes*), point here (to the YES picture). If you hear nothing (shake your head *no*), point here (to the NO picture)". Most four-year-old children can understand the basic instructions after a few repetitions and examples. This test has been administered successfully with some hearing-impaired children as young as three years of age.

Demonstrate the task. In initial trials, present *all* speech sounds without visible cues. This can be achieved by covering your mouth, nose, and the lower part of your face with a slanted card, or an embroidery hoop fitted with acoustically porous cloth (see figure 4.6). Point to your ear, say "listen", obscure your mouth, produce the strong vowel /ɑ/, and uncover your mouth immediately. (Produce the /ɑ/ with a loud voice near the child to ensure detection.) If the child does not immediately point to the YES picture, move his/her hand to the YES picture. After the child points, repeat the /ɑ/ sound, and wait for the appropriate pointing response. Next, cover your mouth, produce the vowel /ɑ/ *silently* (without voice), and uncover your mouth. Most children will immediately point to NO. If the child points to YES, however, say "listen again", cover your mouth, produce the vowel /ɑ/ with no sound, and uncover your mouth. The child should point to NO. Finally, present the vowel /ɑ/ with sound or no sound for several more trials, requiring the child to point to the correct picture each time.

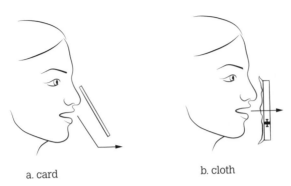

a. card   b. cloth

Figure 4.6 **Cover your mouth with either (a) a card or (b) an embroidery hoop fitted with porous cloth. The nose and lower part of the face must be covered to mask visible articulation**

Occasionally present long sequences of each test item, even four or five in a row. The purpose is to show that this might occur. That is, the child may be required to point to YES or NO repeatedly. You may even present an extremely long sequence as a game, so that the child can demonstrate confidence. Some children enjoy continuously pointing to YES to show you they really are paying attention.

After about a minute of this activity, most children will understand the task, that is, listen when you cover your mouth and respond when you uncover it, regardless of whether or not you produced sound. If the child continues to misunderstand the instructions, you may try substituting a tactile vibrator, returning to the regular listening system after the task is understood. (See Appendix 2 for more information about perception of speech patterns through a vibro-tactile system.)

Conduct the test. When you are confident that the child understands the task, introduce other vowels and consonants in random order. Speak all consonants as *continuants* without an accompanying vowel (e.g., say /vvvvv/, not "vee" or "vuh"). Present each item at least once, preferably twice if you have time, to confirm previous responses. You should also present "no sound" frequently, always marking the child's response to the absence of sound (Schery & Peters 2003). If the child ever responds YES when you present no sound, repeat the instructions, contrasting a loud /ɑ/ with *silence*. Continue testing only after the child responds reliably to this pair. If confusion persists, check the listening system and/or the test environment for unwanted audible noise.

This speech-sound detection test should take approximately 10 minutes. When you have finished testing, look at the pattern of responses (see figure 4.7). Ideally, a hearing-impaired child will detect most speech sounds most of the time, provided the personal listening system has been programmed/mapped appropriately. In reality, however, hearing-impaired children will differ in their ability to detect speech sounds. Some common response patterns include:

- detecting all speech sounds
- detecting most sounds but not voiceless fricatives
- detecting most vowels but few consonants
- detecting only strong central vowels, such as /ɑ/
- detecting no speech sounds. (If this happens, try to diagnose/solve this problem before you proceed.)

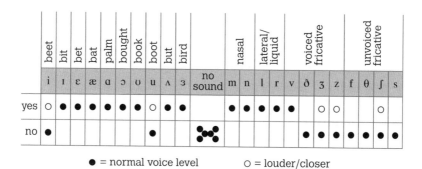

● = normal voice level ○ = louder/closer

Figure 4.7 **A child's detection responses to speech sounds (adapted from Erber 1982)**

As mentioned, some children will be able to detect only a few speech sounds (e.g., mainly vowels) when they listen through their hearing aids. Although their hearing aids are powerful, these children may suffer from frequent colds and/or allergies (with middle ear effusion/fluid and associated conductive hearing loss) that shift their hearing sensitivity beyond the prescribed output of the hearing aids. Their ability to detect speech sounds may even fluctuate from day to day.

Adaptive procedures

After examining the child's auditory responses, re-test using adaptive strategies. This means trying to discover any *special* listening conditions that help the child detect speech sounds that could not be detected under *typical* conditions. For example, speak louder, increase the duration of speech sounds, or sit closer to the child as you speak each vowel and consonant. You may also try different programming/mapping options, or an alternative listening system.

Note your own communication behavior as you *adapt* your speech during this test, that is, write down what you did to help the child detect particular speech sounds. If/when you repeat a similar detection task, you can compare the error patterns and strategies used to overcome the difficulty. For example, if you discovered during previous testing that increasing voice level helped the child to detect your speech, then you know one way to reduce the child's speech-sound detection difficulties. Later, you may discover better solutions, such as decreasing distance, reducing room noise, or modifying/improving the child's listening system.

Some examiners also ask the child to *identify* (repeat) the speech sounds from GASP! Subtest 1, that is, you may ask the child to repeat each speech sound that you present. This is a simple way to quickly obtain additional auditory information. For example, when you ask the child to "Say what I say!" the child may:

- identify the spoken sound correctly = both detection and identification
- respond but identify the spoken sound incorrectly = detection. The incorrect response may indicate which speech features can be identified
- not respond when no sound is presented = correct detection of silence
- respond when no sound is presented ("false positive") = detection of background noise?
- not respond to spoken sound = detection difficulty.

The detection results from GASP! Subtest 1 can be used to place children into two general categories. If most of the vowel and consonant sounds can be detected without difficulty, it is reasonable to go on to assess the child's ability to identify words (GASP! Subtest 2). If little or nothing can be detected, however, it is not appropriate to proceed until you have investigated and resolved the child's speech-audibility difficulty.

GASP! SUBTEST 2: AUDITORY IDENTIFICATION OF WORDS

The purpose of GASP! Subtest 2 is to describe the child's ability to identify common words. We want to know if the child can:

- perceive frequency qualities or intensity patterns only
- perceive words with few/many syllables
- identify words with/without a need for adaptive procedures such as repetition, clarification, context, visible cues.

GASP! Subtest 2 is based on the Children's Auditory Test (CAT) (Erber & Alencewicz 1976), which later was expanded to form the Monosyllable, Trochee, Spondee test (MTS or MonSTr) (Erber & Witt 1977). This approach to auditory assessment has also been used in other tests (e.g., ESP: Moog & Geers 1990; EARS: Allum et al., 2000).

Standard test procedure

Stimulus items. A set of 12 word pictures (common nouns) are typically used in this test. This is a convenient number of pictures for placement before the child. If a young child cannot name all the pictures in the set that you have chosen, substitute pictures of more familiar words before testing.

Place three word pictures, from each of four different stress-pattern categories, in front of the child. These may appear on individual picture cards, or on a large piece of paper. You may color-code the stress-pattern categories, for example, red = monosyllables, yellow = trochees (two syllables with stress on the first syllable), green = spondees (two equally stressed syllables), blue = tri-syllables. Arrange the words from each stress-pattern category in a column headed by a descriptive symbol, and separate the columns of test words clearly (see figure 4.8).

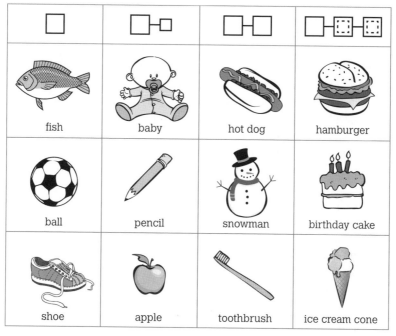

Figure 4.8 **Some pictures used to assess word identification (adapted from Erber 1982)**

Introduce the words. Introduce the test by pointing to a picture (e.g., *ball*) and ask the child "What is this?" with both auditory and visual cues for speech available. The child should say "ball". Then you should say "ball" as you tap the picture once. Hold up one finger and point to your ear to indicate one sound (syllable). Do the same for all one-syllable words. Then gesture generally to all of the pictures in that column to indicate that all of the words are produced with the same sound pattern. If the child does not seem to understand, lightly tap the child's hand or ear once as you speak each word to indicate they all contain one syllable.

Indicate syllable patterns. Follow the same general procedure for the other columns of words, and indicate the appropriate syllable pattern in each case. Eventually the child will understand that each column of words is associated with the symbol at the top. That is, all of the words in a column are produced with a particular syllable pattern. Show the child that there are four different word groups.

Verify word familiarity. If the child cannot name a picture, or names it differently (e.g., says "ice-cream" when you point to *ice-cream cone*), either quickly teach the correct name for the object that is depicted, or substitute a different word picture with the same syllable pattern. The child must be able to name all the pictures correctly before you begin testing. If a child's spoken label for a particular picture contains gross distortions (such as "pence" for *pencil*), try to correct the speech to ensure the child knows the correct syllable pattern, or substitute another word picture.

Practice. After the child has named all of the words, give some general practice as follows. When the child is ready, say one of the test words with both auditory and visual cues, for example, "Show me ... toothbrush." Then shrug your shoulders, gesture, and say, "Where?" (indicating that you want the child to point to a picture). If the child does not point immediately, move the child's finger to the correct picture. Then gradually eliminate the phrase "Show me..." to clarify the listening task. A child who perceives only intensity patterns may identify "Show me ... shoe" as the pattern of a three-syllable word. Instead, wait until the child is ready, say "shoe" alone, gesture, and ask the child to point to a picture. Soon, the child will learn to point to each picture reliably when you name it in isolation with both auditory and visual cues. The aims of practice are to familiarize the child with the general test procedure and the location of the pictures, and to become familiar with the child's typical speed of response.

Conduct the test. Now you are ready to begin the actual test. Tell the child that you will say a word with your mouth covered. Then:

- cover your mouth (as shown in figure 4.6)
- say one of the test words
- uncover your mouth
- wait for the child to point.

Begin by speaking a long word that should be relatively easy to identify, such as *birthday cake*. The response will suggest whether the child can perceive frequency cues or only syllable patterns. If the child instantly points to the *birthday cake* picture, it is likely that many other test words will be identified. If the child points to *hamburger* or *ice-cream cone*, at least syllable patterns can be identified correctly. If the child points to a one- or two-syllable word, however, you may have doubts about the child's ability to identify simple words by listening alone. After initially presenting an "easy" test word (e.g., *birthday cake*), present all other words in a random order.

Indicate the child's response to each stimulus word by placing a dot (•) in the appropriate box of the matrix shown in figure 4.9. Present each word twice, or even three times, if responses to a given word vary – although always present all test words the *same* number of times.

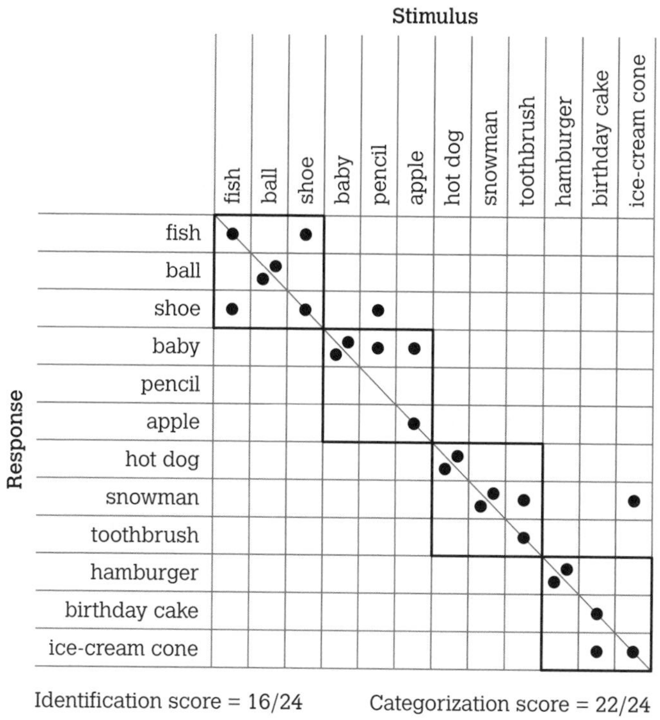

Figure 4.9 **A child's word-identification responses. Each word was presented twice (adapted from Erber 1982)**

Eliminate visible cues. It is important to ensure your eye/head movements do not convey the spoken syllable pattern of a word. To determine if the child is responding to visible movement cues, cover your mouth and present an artificial word like "ball-ball", producing voice only during the first syllable. If the child points to a two-syllable word, you may conclude that your sound pattern is being ignored and instead the child is responding to your eye, head, or facial movements. The challenge is to encourage *listening* rather than *looking* at you for speech information. If the child continues to respond to your eye movements, stop moving your eyes, cover the child's eyes as you produce each test word, or sit beside/behind the child as you administer the test.

Assign scores. You may assign "scores" to responses as they appear in the matrix. The diagonal line indicates the intersection of each identical stimulus and response. Therefore dots that appear on the diagonal line show the number of words identified correctly. The child's *identification* score is the number of dots on this line divided by the total number of words presented.

The four heavily outlined boxes denote occasions where your spoken stimulus and the child's response have the same syllable pattern. Dots that appear in these boxes indicate the number of words categorized correctly by pattern. The child's *categorization* score is the number of dots in the four boxes divided by the total number of words presented. This word-identification subtest takes about 15 minutes. When you are finished, examine the child's response pattern and note that:

- some children will confidently identify most spoken words
- some can identify only a few words reliably (usually those with more syllables)
- others will be able to categorize most words reliably, but not identify them
- still others will be able to distinguish reliably only between one- and three-syllable words
- a few children may respond randomly.

Adaptive procedures

After examining the child's response pattern (e.g., figure 4.9), administer the test again using a variety of adaptive strategies. For example, you may simply repeat a word with no change, increase your voice level, elongate vowels, exaggerate diphthongs, carefully articulate consonants, pause between syllables, and/or produce spondees (compound words like *toothbrush*) with very equal stress. If any of these modifications improve the child's auditory performance, note the methods used and, in particular, whether repetition alone was an effective strategy. Two children may produce identical response patterns, but one child may respond confidently on the first presentation, while the other requires three or four presentations. Also note if a child fails to identify a word, even after you repeat and clarify many times (see Erber 1992a).

You may encounter a child who has great difficulty recognizing the number of syllables in a word. If so, try re-testing while covering the two middle columns. This means that the child must only compare one- and three-syllable words. You may discover that the child can now classify words easily, and identify some of them. Even with this limited set, however, a few children will not be able to categorize words and will respond randomly. If this happens, either the child cannot count syllables or recognize sound patterns, did not understand the instructions, or the child's personal listening system is not working properly.

GASP! SUBTEST 3: AUDITORY COMPREHENSION OF SENTENCES

A sentence is constructed according to rules of word order (syntax), and word meanings (semantics). Thus sentence comprehension usually involves more than merely perception of individual words. An older child may use an accumulated knowledge of language (syntax, semantics, speech-sound sequences) to fill in the parts of a sentence that are not heard clearly. A younger child with less knowledge of language may not be able to compensate for perceptual limitations in this way, and may be unable to decode sentences that are spoken at a normal conversational rate. A test of sentence comprehension, therefore, evaluates more than auditory *perception*. It also evaluates many aspects of the child's ability to process spoken language.

To demonstrate comprehension of a spoken sentence, the child must respond in a way that differs from simple repetition of the sentence, but is related to the sentence in a meaningful way. You may use requests, instructions, or questions to evaluate sentence comprehension. If you use requests or instructions, the child may require much more time to perform the response task than you needed to speak the request or instruction. In contrast, *questions* sample a child's sentence-comprehension ability efficiently. Questions are an important component of spoken communication. Many years ago, a question–answer format was developed to evaluate communication by telephone and radio (Fletcher 1929), and to test hearing (Hudgins et al., 1947). Several speech perception tests for children now include questions as test items (Butt & Chreist 1968; Ludvigsen 1974; Allum et al., 2000). You can construct many question-based tasks to evaluate auditory comprehension. These tasks are likely to have different degrees of "conversational naturalness". While natural test sentences are preferred in order to obtain results that reflect daily communication, it can be difficult to create realistic test questions that can be used across different children and situations.

Sentence-comprehension materials differ in conversational naturalness

Artificial context: The context is artificially limited, and/or the question–response sequence is not conversational. For example, the child looks at pictures of unrelated objects in a closed set (small white cat, big black cat, small gray dog, big brown dog). The adult asks, "What color is the big cat?"

Instructional context: The child's response is not restricted by a closed set, but the question–response sequence is only moderately conversational. For example, the adult asks, "What is two plus three?" or "How many sides does a triangle have?"

Conversational context: The question–response sequence is conversational. For example, the adult asks, "How old is your little brother?" or "What did you have for lunch?" It can be difficult, however, to create conversational questions that are not specific to each child and situation.

GASP! Subtest 3 includes simple questions that a teacher might ask a young child. Previous results suggest that children who are able to identify words by listening alone often can also answer some of these spoken questions by listening alone. Conversely, most children who are unable to identify words by listening alone will be unable to answer questions by listening alone.

Standard test procedure

This auditory comprehension subtest uses 10 simple questions that include the question forms *what, where, when, how many*, and so forth. The test is given in an open-set format without related objects or pictorial prompts. You simply instruct the child, "I'm going to ask some questions. Please tell me the answers."

Introduce task. Speak several sample questions (see figure 4.10) with both auditory and visual cues to familiarize the child with the task. For example, ask (without gesturing), "How many fingers do you have?" If the child fails to answer correctly, repeat the question with both auditory and visual cues. If the answer is still not forthcoming, repeat again, and exaggerate the acoustic pattern (e.g., stress the words *How many*). If this attempt fails, repeat the question with extreme clarity (and/or with gestures) to help the child respond correctly (e.g., wiggle your fingers). If the child requires this much help to answer a simple question with both auditory and visual cues, however, it is not likely that the child will be able to answer similar questions by *listening* alone when you begin actual testing. Regardless, write the answer on the response form (figure 4.10), and proceed to the next two sample questions. If the child still seems unsure of what to do (after you have presented these samples with both auditory and visual cues), you may create a few more questions for practice and present the instructions again, being careful not to ask (at this time) any of the 10 questions that form the actual comprehension test.

Test. When the child understands that you will ask questions and expect answers, tell the child it is time to listen. Cover your mouth (see figure 4.6), and ask a test question. Then uncover your mouth, and wait for an answer. For example, you may ask, "What is your teacher's name?" If the child answers correctly, give a mark (•) for a correct answer and proceed to the next question (see figure 4.10).

Sentence (question)	Response	Comment	Rep	Aud
1 (What is your name?)	Richard	difficult	4	
2 What color are your shoes?	blue	shoes > chair	2	●
3 How many people are in your family?	4	confident	1	●
4 (Where is your hearing aid)/cochlear implant?	points to ear		5	
5 When is your birthday?	November 22	confident	1	●
6 What is your teacher's name?	Miss Powell		2	●
7 (What number comes after seven?)	4, 8, 9, etc.	"comes after"	9	
8 How many legs does an elephant have?	4	confident	1	●
9 Where do you live?	S. Kingsville	no problem	1	●
10 How old are (you?)	13	you > we	6	

Clarification (Gesture) (A-V)   Score = $\frac{6}{10}$

Practice
How many fingers do you have?   Where is your mouth?   What color is the table?

Figure 4.10 **A child's sentence-comprehension responses (adapted from Erber 1982)**

Adaptive procedures

The purpose of adaptive testing is to find out how well the child responds to simple questions, and to discover which adaptive procedures are needed to elicit appropriate answers. When you ask a question (e.g., "What is your teacher's name?"), the child may respond incorrectly, or not at all. If this happens, tell the child you will say it again, cover your mouth, and repeat the question. If the answer is "Elizabeth!" (sister's name), the child is aware you are asking for a name. Try saying "teacher's" a little louder. If the child still responds incorrectly, you may elongate the vowel /i/ in teacher's, exaggerate the affricate /tʃ/, or pause briefly between syllables. Alternatively, try presenting the confused word alone, without sentence context, and then repeat the entire question (see Erber & McMahon 1976; Nittrouer & Boothroyd 1990; Eisenberg et al., 2002).

You may simply ask the child, "What did I say?" and request an *identification* response (in this case, the child is likely to respond, "You said, 'What is your sister's name?'"). You can prompt the child with your mouth covered. For example, after the child responds "Elizabeth", say, "No, that is your *sister's* name. What is your *teacher's* name?" You can contrast the two confused words: "You said your *sister's* name; I said your *teacher's* name". If you provide additional information like this without visible cues and receive a correct response, the child receives "credit" for auditory comprehension of the sentence (see figure 4.10).

If the child does not respond correctly after many attempts to obtain an answer to a spoken question, as described above, you may conclude that the correct response will not be forthcoming through listening alone. It is important, however, not to give up on listening too soon. You can try repeating the question, but uncover your mouth briefly as you say the key word *teacher's*. The child may now respond correctly to your question ("Miss Powell"). If so, write the child's response, but do not give a mark (•), because visible cues were required. Instead, draw a circle around the word *teacher's* to indicate that you spoke it with visible cues.

Similarly, if you emphasize a particular word(s) to aid the child's auditory comprehension, indicate this by underlining. If you need to present a question several times to obtain a correct answer, write down the number of repetitions required. Follow this same procedure with all test questions.

Try to help the child answer each question correctly *without* allowing lipreading. If you need to provide visible cues to compensate for auditory difficulty, the child cannot receive credit for answering the question. Instead, your goal is to help the child comprehend the greatest number of sentences (questions) by *listening* alone, using whatever acoustic strategies you can create and apply. You must, however, continually assess whether your persistence is stressful. Usually, if you demonstrate by your relaxed manner that a lack of immediate success does not worry *you*, the child will be encouraged to continue listening.

The child's score is the number of questions answered correctly (out of 10) with only acoustic cues provided. The results will also include a detailed record of the various communication strategies you used to help the child succeed. After administering GASP! Subtest 3, you will know:

- how well the child can comprehend simple sentences (questions) by listening alone
- a variety of useful clarification techniques for facilitating auditory communication and learning.

With this adaptive test, two children may obtain the same numerical "score", yet one child answers all questions easily without hesitation, and the other requires six repetitions and several clarification strategies. A learning goal for the first child may be to extend auditory comprehension skills, for example, to include more complex language in daily conversation. For the second child, a learning goal may be to reduce the amount of adaptive participation and effort by the parent or teacher.

APPLICATIONS OF ADAPTIVE HEARING ASSESSMENT

Most auditory speech-perception tests are scored as the percentage of spoken items correctly identified. This score specifies not only the proportion of test items that the child can hear and identify (e.g., 30 per cent) but also how much the child *cannot* identify (70 per cent in this case). Most parents and teachers want to know how to communicate the spoken items the child apparently cannot identify.

Adaptive Hearing Assessment is an alternative method for describing a child's ability to perceive spoken words, phrases, or sentences. If a test item cannot be identified, the examiner *adapts* to the child's error by changing the way the item is presented (see sentence-comprehension procedure above). The adult repeats, clarifies and provides context or visible cues until the child is successful. The results describe conditions under which the child can identify the test material. Parents and teachers can use this information to plan instruction and to communicate successfully.

Table 4.1 **Adaptive strategies can be applied before, during, or after presentation of each stimulus item**

Before	adult speaks a related word ("Christmas" > *wreath*) child asks a related question ("What happened when the cat meowed?" > *The dog made an angry noise*) (Erber 1992b; Flynn & Dowell 1999)
During	meaningful context visible cues for speech fewer response alternatives
After	repeat clarify modify

This general method of assessment is a form of diagnostic teaching, in which instruction is integrated with assessment. You can include adaptive methods whenever you administer an auditory speech-perception test – whether or not you use the GASP! materials as previously described.

It is not difficult to create a speech perception test that follows the common conversational sequence shown in figure 4.2. Any set of words or sentences can be presented in an adaptive manner. You can use items from a standard speech perception test like the WIPI (Ross & Lerman 1979) or NU-CHIPS (Elliott & Katz 1980), or simply create a list of common words from the child's home or school environment (e.g., *dish, apple, paint, teacher, door*). The general procedure is summarized below:

4   obtain or create a list of test words
5   speak a test word (without visible cues)

6   if the child identifies the word, proceed to the next word
7   if the child responds incorrectly, however, adapt to the child's error (e.g., repeat, clarify, provide context/visible cues, etc.)
8   when the child responds correctly, note the communication condition under which word identification occurred, and proceed to the next item.

Cumulative word-identification results

What follows are some examples of how the adaptive assessment procedure is applied. A 14-year-old boy listened through his behind-the-ear hearing aids to a female examiner who spoke 25 words from the WIPI test. He identified 12 of 25 words (48 per cent) correctly following their original (O) presentation (see figure 4.11). When the remaining 13 words were repeated (R), he was able to hear and identify five more words. Successive presentations with clarification (C), sentence context (S), and sentence context with visible cues (SAV) enabled the boy to identify progressively more words.

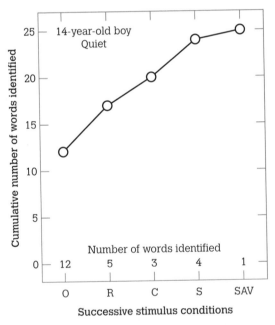

Figure 4.11 **Cumulative word-identification results as a function of successive methods of presentation**

The results are shown as the *cumulative* number of words identified following each successive method of presentation: O, R, C, S, SAV. The boy eventually identified all 25 test words.

Word-identification in noise

Children must communicate in different environmental conditions at home and at school. Communicating in background noise can be tiring for both the child and the communication partner.

An eight-year-old girl listened through her behind-the-ear hearing aids to a female examiner who spoke sets of 25 words from the WIPI test under three background conditions: quiet, +15 dB S/N, and 0 dB S/N. Figure 4.12 shows the cumulative number of words identified correctly as a function of successive methods of presentation in each background condition. The girl identified (nearly) all test words in all conditions, but she achieved this much more quickly and easily when listening in quiet.

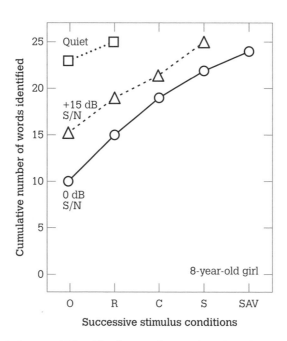

Figure 4.12 **Cumulative word-identification results as a function of successive methods of presentation under three environmental conditions**

Benefit of an FM system

Audiologists generally recommend that hearing-impaired children use wireless FM systems when they listen in noisy school classrooms. A 10-year-old girl listened to a female examiner who spoke sets of 25 words from the WIPI test in a moderate amount of background noise (0 dB S/N). Figure 4.13 shows the cumulative number of test words identified as a function of listening condition (binaural behind-the-ear hearing aids, FM system). The girl eventually identified all test words under both listening conditions, but she reached this level much more quickly and easily when listening through the FM system.

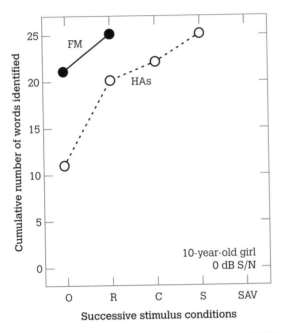

Figure 4.13 **Cumulative word-identification results when a child listened in noise under two conditions (own hearing aids, wireless FM system)**

INTERPRETING ADAPTIVE HEARING ASSESSMENT RESULTS

The results of adaptive hearing assessment specify the conditions (e.g., repetition, clarification, context) under which a child can identify test items. Instead of describing hearing for speech as a per cent–correct score, the child's listening behavior is described in terms of:

- the conditions under which the child responds correctly
- the child's confidence and willingness to respond
- the child's strengths and weaknesses in facilitating good communication
- the amount of examiner effort and creativity required.

The results obtained from administration of the three GASP! subtests provide general information about the child's current auditory abilities. These findings will suggest directions for extending the child's listening skills. For example:

- the child may be able to detect some speech sounds but not others, and may benefit from reprogramming the personal listening system
- the child may be able to identify some words, but respond with less confidence or accuracy to words that contain only one syllable or high-frequency consonants, and may benefit from listening practice
- the child may be able to answer most simple questions, and may benefit from conversational experience.

Through repeated testing and interaction, you will learn which adaptive communication strategies are most effective for the child. Parents and other communication partners can use this information to adapt their own communication to suit the child.

In most cases, the per cent–correct score obtained for the original (O) presentation of test materials underestimates the child's potential for auditory communication. Many children can obtain much higher speech detection, identification, or comprehension "scores" if the test conditions are modified sufficiently, and appropriate adaptive strategies are applied. Examples of adaptive strategies include:

- repeating
- increasing voice level
- speaking more slowly
- articulating more precisely
- emphasizing speech sounds, syllables, or key words
- pausing between syllables or words
- providing supplementary information (e.g., "It's the name of an animal")
- employing acoustic prompts (e.g., "It's not a bird")
- contrasting your spoken stimulus with the child's (incorrect) response
- requesting a lower-level response (e.g., "What did I say?" while assessing sentence comprehension)
- simplifying or rephrasing a sentence
- providing visible cues.

The results of adaptive auditory assessment can be summarized easily in reports to parents and teachers, suggesting strategies they can use when communicating with the child. For example:

- benefits from using a wireless FM system
- benefits from clear speech, so articulate carefully with a slower-than-normal rate
- often requires repetition, so cooperation and patience are necessary
- benefits from linguistic/conversational/situational context
- benefits from visible cues for speech.

Regular assessments with an adaptive procedure can be used to describe a child's progress as a listener over a period of time. Each time a test is administered, the examiner is likely to speak and apply communication strategies in a different way, according to the child's immediate needs. Typically, the child's reliance on the speaker's effort and creativity will diminish over time, as the child gains skill as a communicator.

SUMMARY

Many speech perception tests have been developed to evaluate a hearing-impaired child's listening skills, but most yield only per cent-correct scores and do not indicate how to help the child during auditory communication. Adaptive hearing assessment (AHA!) is an approach to auditory testing that both measures communication ability and specifies:

1 the conditions under which the child achieves best auditory communication
2 the amount and type of cooperation, clarification, and creativity that the communication partner must provide to reach this level.

The features of adaptive hearing assessment are that:

- it may be used with any standard test or any list of words/sentences that you create
- it requires spoken responses from the child
- it may be used to compare the effects of different listening conditions (e.g., quiet versus noise; hearing aids versus an FM system)
- it may be used to measure a change in performance over time (in terms of reduced need for adaptive behavior by the adult).

The GASP! can be used to evaluate a child's auditory speech perception at three levels:

1 speech-sound detection
2 word identification
3 sentence (question) comprehension.

During GASP! testing, the adult applies adaptive strategies to help the child succeed as a listener. The results indicate how auditory communication can be improved.

CHAPTER 5

Listening and learning

After a young hearing-impaired child has received hearing aids or cochlear implants, the first listening goals are usually development of awareness and attention to sound, and participation in unstructured vocal interaction. Over the following months and years, the child starts to acquire an auditory basis for language and communication, and learns to interpret acoustic details in speech. By school age, many hearing-impaired children are able to use spoken language to access information and develop social relationships.

EARLY CHILDHOOD

The years from birth to three are an optimal time for listening and learning. Key features of communication during early childhood include the following:
- the distance between the adult communicator and the child is usually short
- most interactions occur in familiar surroundings
- the main communication partners are motivated to help the child learn.

In a typical early childhood learning program, the therapist models communication and teaching behavior for parents and shows them how to support the young child's auditory development. The therapist shows the parents how to incorporate listening experience into daily activities (Simmons-Martin & Rossi 1990; Estabrooks 1994; Simser 1999; Cole & Flexer 2011). Parents are encouraged to follow natural patterns of spoken interaction with the child as closely as possible. For example, parents are shown how to:
- integrate listening into daily routines and experiences
- talk about the child's immediate interests and activities
- repeat familiar play songs and rhymes
- vary sound patterns as with a child who has normal hearing
- speak with age-appropriate language and content
- talk naturally without exaggerated mouth movements
- use natural, appropriate facial expressions.

Parents learn to encourage an infant's babbling, play-talk, and expressive jargon as part of normal development. The parents draw the child's attention to naturally occurring sounds in and near the home (e.g., a door closing, a car in the driveway, rain on the roof, a dog barking). For example, "Listen! I hear Jeff's doggie! Let's go and see his doggie!"

AUDITORY SKILLS CHECKLIST

Educators have provided checklists of auditory skills to help parents and therapists describe a young child's level of development and to specify listening goals (Franz et al., 2004; Stredler-Brown 2010). Activity guides and training materials for each skill have also been produced (Romanik 2008).

Desirable listening skills include:
- awareness and attention to sound
- locating and identifying the source of a sound
- hearing at a distance from the source of a sound
- perception of prosody, voice pitch, emotion
- memory for spoken sequences
- listening in background noise.

For example, a parent may learn to:
- speak the child's name to gain attention, rather than relying on vision or touch
- associate the sounds of speech with all experiences, toys, and play activities: /b/: *bus*; /p/: *push*; /r/: *roll*
- associate sounds with animals and toys: *cow* = "moo", *sheep* = "baa", *cat* = "meow", *dog* = "woof"
- incorporate repetitive acoustic patterns into daily communication and play: "up-up-up!"
- repeat common phrases in their appropriate situational contexts: "yum-yum", "all gone", "thank you", "bye-bye"
- show the child when a response is expected
- pause to allow the child time to respond
- provide praise or a reward for good listening.

Listening activities progress from easier to more difficult tasks, including:
- simple > more complex rhythmic patterns
- louder > softer speech sounds
- discrimination between (for example) central (/ɑ/) < > front/back (/i, u/) vowels, voiced (/b/) < > voiceless (/p/) stop consonants, voiced (/v/) < > voiceless (/f/) fricative consonants
- identification of words, at first in small closed sets with few alternatives, and later in open sets without limiting context

- gradual increase of the child's attention span to include longer units of spoken language such as phrases and sentences
- gradual increase of the child's auditory memory to include more than one word, phrase, or sentence
- conversation in quiet > conversation during play and social interaction.

The child learns to listen to whispered speech, speech produced by different people, sounds at a distance (e.g., that originate in the next room or outside), musical rhythms and melodies, and speech in a small amount of background noise (e.g., a heater or air conditioner). Sessions are both instructive and diagnostic. Informal "testing" during listening activities and spoken interaction with the child indicate current needs and suggest future auditory goals.

Listening skills can be placed into general categories to form new dimensions or "layers" of the stimulus-response matrix shown previously in figure 3.3 including:

- speaker location (distance/angle of the sound source)
- speech quality (syllable pattern, pitch, prosody, clarity)
- message complexity (number of modifiers, phrases, instructions)
- background competition (noise, echo, auditory/visual distraction).

Factors that can affect ease of listening

The ease or difficulty of any listening task is related to: the size of the "response set", number of syllables, acoustic clarity of the stimulus items, speech rate, linguistic complexity, familiarity of the items, context, situation/environment, and availability of visible cues (Schery & Peters 2003; Kent 2004).

Adults have used the Situ-Action training procedure (Erber & Lamb 1995) to discover how seven key factors interact to influence ease of speech communication: the child's hearing ability, vision ability, personal listening system, distance between communicators, surrounding environment, partner's speech clarity, and complexity of conversation. The latter four factors are similar to the dimensions included in most listening skill checklists. They can be modified in many ways to make communication easier.

OLDER CHILDREN

For older children, speech communication is a regular part of daily life, both at home and at school. The child learns, plays, and communicates with other children using speech and hearing. Friendships and social relationships become very important.

The school environment presents new challenges. For example:

- the distance between communicators in a classroom is often greater than at home

- the classroom may be noisy and distracting
- the child needs to acquire information from teachers
- an FM listening system may be used to improve the teacher's audibility.

Adults must continue to help increase the child's listening skills in order to cope with these increased auditory requirements and to learn from spoken language.

After a child's listening skills have been assessed, goals will be established for continued auditory development. There are several adaptive communication methods that can be used to provide ongoing listening experience including:

- natural conversation
- shared experience
- specific listening activity.

Adaptive approaches to auditory communication

Natural conversation

- The adult speaks to the child in a natural manner in the context of daily life.
- Listening tasks are derived from any box in the stimulus-response matrix (e.g., narrative comprehension).
- The adult adapts to the child's responses with listening tasks selected from any other box in the matrix.

Shared experience

- The adult selects the topic and content related to a recent shared experience.
- The adult presents a "closed-set" identification task.
- The adult adapts to the child's responses with listening tasks selected from neighboring boxes in the matrix (e.g., word/sentence identification and comprehension).

Specific listening activity

- The adult prepares materials and plans a listening activity according to the child's need for specific practice.
- The adult presents a closed- or open-set listening task.
- Attention is directed to a particular listening skill, usually within a single box in the matrix (e.g., phrase discrimination).

A NATURAL CONVERSATION APPROACH

Typically, when hearing-impaired children listen to an adult, they also watch the adult's face and mouth. Face-to-face interaction is part of normal language development and social bonding. An adult's facial expression conveys linguistic information such as (mis)understanding, (dis)agreement, and emotional state. Mouth movements convey important vowel and consonant information. Most people with *normal* hearing rely on visible oral and facial cues to maintain conversational fluency in noise or other difficult listening conditions.

There are many occasions, however, when a child communicates without direct face-to-face contact. For example:

- a parent's face may not be visible when speaking to the child while cleaning the floor
- a teacher's face may not be visible when she turns her head to respond to another child
- a young friend's face may not be visible while climbing a ladder in the playground.

A hearing-impaired child can benefit from listening when the visible components of speech are obscured, intermittent, or simply not available. Practitioners of the auditory-verbal approach recommend listening without lipreading as a way to stimulate the child's auditory system, and develop complex auditory processing abilities (Beebe 1953; Pollack 1970). Research indicates that a primarily auditory-only strategy can facilitate the growth of a child's spoken language (Rhoades & Chisholm 2000; Rhoades 2006).

Parents and other communication partners can provide listening experiences to a hearing-impaired child by conversing during most daily activities. This is done by simply talking to the child about what is happening, providing listening experience without specifically directing attention to the movements and positions of your mouth (Beebe 1953; Pollack 1970, 1984; Erber 1982; Estabrooks 1994; Simser 1993, 1999). It is not necessary to cover your mouth, although you may do so. Instead, you may stand behind, or sit beside the child as you work and play together.

Another option is to speak while clearly visible to the child, if that is your usual orientation during a particular activity. Simply obscure your mouth when you come to particular words, phrases, or sentences, and encourage the child to listen. After a small amount of practice, this type of listening "game" should neither bother the child, nor disrupt your communication.

Children with similar pure-tone thresholds are likely to differ in their ability to hear speech (Erber 1974b). Some children hear speech so well they can easily engage in conversation without watching the speaker. Others are far more dependent on visible cues. They may have insufficient listening experience and/or poor auditory processing skills. Most children are able to improve their ability to listen if they receive regular listening experience with enjoyable auditory communication activities.

Many children quickly improve their auditory skills (and rely less on visible cues) when they realize that you typically talk to them about what is happening or what they are doing such as visiting grandma, feeding the dog, or having a bath. A child may reasonably expect you to speak only a limited range of words and phrases in that context. Each situational context restricts what you will say, limits the child's expectations, and increases auditory understanding. For example, if you speak to a child while observing a small furry animal, you are more likely to say "What color is the mouse?" than "Aunt Carol's in the house!"

To ensure success, the goal for each listening task needs to be based on previously achieved auditory skills. New listening tasks should either consolidate, or extend the child's abilities, but they should not be too far out of reach. In choosing appropriate tasks, remember that:

- an open-set listening task with unlimited alternatives is more difficult than a closed-set task with few alternatives
- some speech sounds are much harder to identify than others
- spoken sentences differ greatly in their linguistic complexity.

Occasionally, spoken interaction with a hearing-impaired child will break down, and the child will respond incorrectly or not at all. When this happens, you will need to apply communication strategies to restore the fluency of conversation. You can find out what the child heard by requesting an identification response (e.g., "What did I say?" or "What did you hear?"). If you request identification responses too often, however, you may disrupt conversations and make the interaction unnatural. Therefore, you must compromise between: (1) helping the child develop a complete sound-based concept of spoken language and (2) maintaining the child's interest in listening.

Do not forget that children with normal hearing acquire (and produce) language forms incompletely at first ("Dada work!"). They eventually learn that they also must supply the less prominent unstressed syllables ("Daddy is going to work!"). When part of a sentence is heard without clarity (e.g., an inaudible syllable or a new word), even a child with normal hearing will rely on the situational and/or linguistic context and "guess" what was said, discovering later whether the interpretation was correct or not.

Applying the natural conversation approach

Example 1: A parent applies the natural conversation approach with a young child who does not regularly respond with spoken language. It is time for breakfast, and the mother of a young child has just placed him in his highchair. She sits beside him and conducts the following "monologue" (most of the child's responses are *non-verbal*): "Are you hungry? Here is your elephant bowl! Put the rice bubbles in the bowl ... Mummy will put some banana on top ... Pour the milk – pour, pour, pour. Here is your spoon. Open wide – chew, chew, chew. You spilled some milk on your chin! Do you want more banana? Yummmm ... all gone! Good boy! Mummy will wipe your face. You can go and play now. Bye bye!"

Example 2: A parent applies the natural conversation approach during a daily activity. A mother of a school-age child is beginning to cook dinner. She starts to boil water and get some ingredients from the cupboard. She tells the child about her plans for dinner and asks for help: "It's time to get ready for dinner. Go and wash your hands." … "We're having spaghetti tonight. Where are the big bowls?" … "You can help – go and get the spaghetti. The box is over there by the fridge!" … "Where is the tomato sauce?" … "Thank you! You're a very good helper!" … "Now give each person a knife, a fork, and a spoon." … "Please go and tell Andrew to stop watching TV, wash his hands, and come in here!"

This is a common occurrence in most families, where daily rituals quickly become familiar to the child. Under these conditions, it should not be difficult for the child to learn to recognize spoken requests. Most home situations and activities provide excellent opportunities for auditory communication (e.g., getting dressed, making the bed, going shopping, playing with toys, baking a cake, digging in the garden, or bath time).

Example 3: A pre-school teacher applies a natural conversation approach during classroom art and craft activities. He provides paper, paint, and brushes, and suggests that a child paint a picture. The teacher sits beside or behind the child, so that the child can hear but not see him, and gives instructions or asks questions. The teacher might suggest what to paint ("Put some pretty red flowers near the house …"), or might suggest how to make new colors ("If you mix blue and yellow together, you will get green! What happens when you mix blue and red?"). The child may follow the teacher's instructions or request clarification.

Some hearing-impaired children respond easily to auditory communication. They do not need to both listen and watch the teacher to understand spoken messages in a familiar context. Other children may turn to the teacher frequently for additional visual information. The teacher may repeat the message while the child is looking and listening, but after the child returns to the task, the teacher will repeat or paraphrase the message so that the child can focus on the sound pattern. Alternatively, the teacher may elaborate without providing visible cues ("The red flowers are beautiful!"). This can be a relatively casual, relaxed activity, which can build confidence in listening.

Example 4: A teacher uses a "barrier game" (Greenspan et al., 1975; Yule 1997) to give a child practice in listening to and comprehending spoken instructions (see figure 5.1). The teacher constructs a simple visual barrier between the child and herself. She then draws a picture or constructs a small toy or object (e.g., with colored pens, blocks, etc.), keeping it hidden from view. Without visible cues, the teacher describes the picture or object step-by-step (sentence-by-sentence). The listening task can be very easy ("Draw a circle") or very difficult ("Put the girl with the green dress in the vegetable garden by the black duck"). The child's task is to listen carefully and use similar materials to replicate the teacher's action, for example, to draw a picture, construct an object, or follow a path that matches the teacher's description (Lloyd et al., 2005).

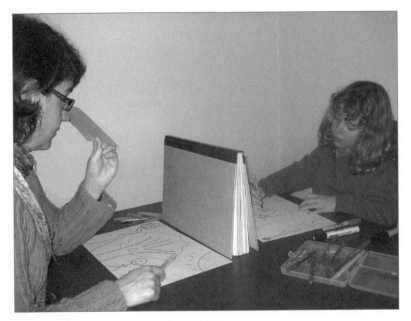

Figure 5.1 **A barrier game**

The teacher can guide the child's behavior by providing acoustic prompts (e.g., "Listen carefully ... the dog is *brown!*"). The teacher should adapt vocabulary and language according to the child's responses and requests for clarification. After the child is finished, the barrier is removed and the child and teacher can compare their work.

Many young hearing-impaired children can sustain attention to this type of activity for a long time. Barrier games are good for increasing a young child's confidence in listening. When the drawings or toys are compared afterwards, the child receives tangible evidence that comprehension has been successful and the spoken instructions were followed accurately.

Example 5: A teacher uses a conversational approach in an arithmetic class while all children are occupied with independent work. In this situation, the teacher goes from child to child and comments on each one's work, or asks questions without visual cues. That is, the teacher stands behind or beside the child and provides instruction, perhaps occasionally pointing or gesturing to the work (see figure 5.2). It is easier for the child to understand the teacher's speech if the context is first established by naming or pointing to the item that will be discussed (e.g., "the second multiplication problem").

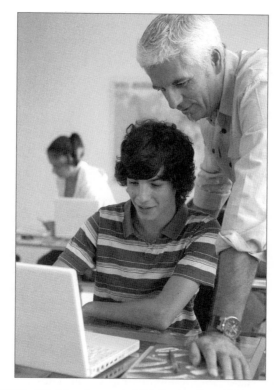

Figure 5.2 **A teacher and child discuss the child's work**

If the child does not initially understand, the teacher may try repeating or clarifying the message. When the child is able to follow the instructions through listening, it is important for the teacher to comment positively ("Good listening!"). This increases confidence in listening alone to acquire information. At first, a child may not be willing to follow a spoken request until there is certainty about what was said. The child may repeatedly ask for clarification. Patiently repeat and encourage listening, especially if the child is motivated and interested. Be supportive – ask the child to "take a chance" and attempt to respond. Indicate that you are not disappointed if at first the child doesn't understand, but that you value any attempt.

Example 6: A parent takes advantage of listening opportunities that occur while the parent and child are at a park, museum, or zoo. The parent may stand behind or beside the child and say, "I see three monkeys!" and continue to talk about the animals while the child watches ("Look, there's a baby monkey!"). Without warning, the parent might ask "Would you like an ice-cream?" to determine if the child can understand a much-anticipated question when spoken out of context. Similar opportunities for casual auditory communication can occur in the home while working together in the garden, cooking in the kitchen, or putting toys away (see figure 5.3).

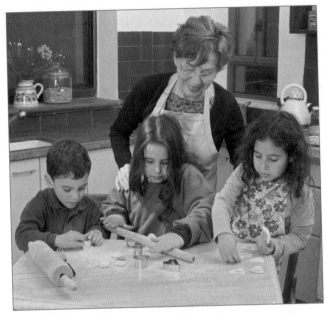

Figure 5.3 **An opportunity for auditory communication**

Example 7: A therapist combines listening practice with natural auditory-visual communication by systematically eliminating visible cues as she speaks. While looking at a map and reviewing geography facts with a child, a therapist may present detailed information in complete sentences, although the child may only be able to identify short phrases through listening alone. In this situation, the therapist can present auditory-visual cues during most of a sentence, but eliminate the visual component when speaking particular words. Thus, in response to the child's question, "Where is Ethiopia?" she might present most of her answer: "Ethiopia is a country in northeast Africa", with both auditory and visual cues, but cover her mouth with her hand as she produces the last few words, thereby requiring the child to *listen* for these key items. Given the topic, the context provided by his question, and the redundancy of the sentence, the child may be able to identify the spoken phrase "northeast Africa", although it contains many weak high-pitched consonants.

Example 8: A parent discusses past and future events and absent objects with an older child. If a child can manage open-set listening with unlimited response alternatives, you can conduct conversations about objects that are not physically present or events/activities that are not currently in progress. You and the child may discuss something that happened previously or will happen in the future. These conversations require the child to possess memory, imagination, reasoning, and/or planning skills. For example, a parent, therapist, or teacher may obscure her mouth and say:

- "Where are your brown shoes? Did you put them by the door? Are they in the bedroom? Go and have a look!"
- "Last week we went to the museum. Do you remember what we saw? It was a big animal. The animal lived a long time ago."
- "Today we are going to bake a chocolate cake. We have flour and sugar. What else do we need? What should we do first? How can we find out?"

Using adaptive strategies in natural conversation

Fluent adult–child conversation depends on comprehension of spoken messages. It is useful to refer to the stimulus-response matrix (see figure 3.4) and to treat each of the tasks (boxes) as a component of *conversation*. Thus, when a misunderstanding occurs during a conversation with a hearing-impaired child, you can apply an appropriate remedial strategy – either simplify the content of your message, or apply a lower-level comprehension, identification, discrimination, or detection task.

For example, while reading a book to a hearing-impaired child with your mouth obscured, you may speak the following sentence: "The little girl said, 'Good afternoon!'" If the child appears confused, you may request identification of the misunderstood sentence, and simply ask the child "What did you hear?" If the child responds, "I think the girl said ... *big extra meal!*", then you might quickly try auditory identification of a key word ("What do you hear when I say ... afternoon?"), or a same–different discrimination activity, comparing the phrases *big extra meal* and *good afternoon*. The child's responses will give you insight into the previous perceptual confusion. This adaptive sequence may be accomplished within about 20 seconds, provided that you and the child are familiar with the procedures.

This process of rapidly shifting between stimulus and response levels may not be successful unless you explain your intent to the child (e.g., "Don't try to answer the question now ... just tell me what I said", or "What was the last word?" or "Do these two words sound the same ...?" or "Can you hear this?"). It is important to help the child understand the difference between (1) real conversation and (2) your persistent analysis and remediation of communication difficulties (meta-communication). You may need to develop a set of simple cues or prompts (e.g., "Time out!") to inform the child that you are going to withdraw from the ongoing conversation for a moment and analyze/practice a part of it instead. This type of instructional behavior might be compared to that of a film director who interrupts a scene to guide the actors regarding an exchange of dialog.

The conversation adaptation cycle

Figure 5.4 summarizes the sequence that an adult may follow during daily conversation with a hearing-impaired child. Begin the process by obscuring your mouth to eliminate visible cues. Then present a statement or question. If the child responds correctly, reward the child's successful comprehension, and resume the conversation through listening alone. If the child continues to comprehend what you say without difficulty, either maintain auditory communication at that level, or adapt to the child's (and your) success by substituting new vocabulary and/or more complex language.

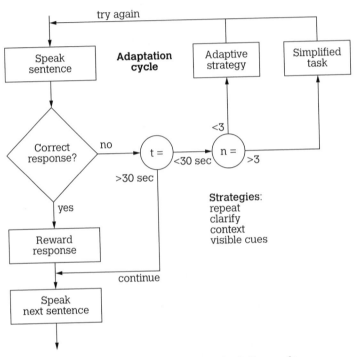

Figure 5.4 **The conversation adaptation cycle**

If, however, the child misunderstands what you say while listening alone, and responds either incorrectly or not at all, you will need to analyze the situation and decide how you will manage it. The child's difficulty may be related either to impaired auditory perception, or to vocabulary or language limitations. You can try a variety of *adaptive* strategies to assist the child with these auditory communication difficulties. Your decision will depend on your experience. Possible strategies include (Erber & Greer 1973; Tye-Murray 1994):

- repeating part or all of what you said
- clarifying your articulation
- emphasizing stress or intonation
- pausing briefly between syllables, words, or phrases

- simplifying the vocabulary
- decreasing the length and complexity of your sentence
- increasing the redundancy of your message
- redefining the context and topic ("The little girl saw her teacher … then what happened?")
- allowing the child to see part or all of what you said.

If you have tried several (e.g., n = 3) adaptive strategies without success, you may simplify the task by asking the child to respond at a lower level (auditory identification: "What did I say?"). After a reasonable amount of time (e.g., t = 30 seconds), you may simply decide to provide visible cues or even to bypass the difficult sentence. You may follow this *adaptation cycle* several times, as you modify a sentence during a conversation, before you determine if the child can comprehend your original message by listening alone.

A SHARED EXPERIENCE APPROACH

Even if a child has considerable hearing and listening ability, parents and teachers must use adaptive procedures to ensure the success of a conversational approach. Adherence to the conversational method requires awareness of the child's listening skills, familiarity with adaptive communication procedures, and conscious control over one's own communication behavior. Initially, some parents and teachers cannot manage all of these factors at the same time. Because they need a more prescribed approach, a simplified listening activity may be preferred.

Nearly anyone can apply auditory communication principles successfully by following the "shared experience" approach. This type of listening activity is a little more formal than the conversational approach just described, but it still retains some components of conversation. The method is based on the "experience story" format developed by Simmons (1968, 1971), after earlier work by Streng et al. (1955) and Groht (1958), and later extended by Golf (1970), Simmons-Martin and Rossi (1990), Easterbrooks and Estes (2007), and others. The original purpose of the method was to help a child associate spoken language with recent home or school experiences.

To use this method, you and the child first need to participate in some sort of shared experience. This can be a planned excursion, such as a visit to your local post office, or something as simple as playing outside (see figure 5.5). After the shared experience, talk about it with the child. You may describe the activity, or you could ask the child to tell you what happened.

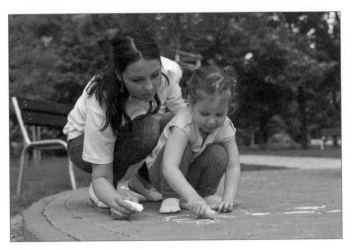

Figure 5.5 **A shared experience approach to auditory communication**

Then write a small set of descriptive sentences and important words or phrases that differ in length, complexity, prosody, vocabulary, etc. to make them relatively easy to identify through hearing alone. The items may be placed in a list (one above the other), or placed on large cards (side-by-side). The degree to which the items must differ acoustically will depend on the child's listening skills and previous experience with similar auditory tasks. Even a child with poor listening and reading skills can participate in this type of activity if the items are made sufficiently different. Experiment with different item types to determine how variations in pattern and content affect listening performance.

Usually, only a small amount of effort is required to create a set of items that differ in the number of syllables, location of major pauses, and content. The set below is a good example of a varied list of items.

A set of items that differ in length and pattern

It rained, but we went outside anyway. (long sentence)

Nick got very wet. (short sentence)

Five birds sat in a tree. They were singing. (two sentences)

.... (nothing)

playground ("spondee" word)

boots (monosyllabic word)

It can sometimes be difficult to select words and/or construct a set of sentences that sound different to a particular hearing-impaired child. Although your written sentences may appear to differ in length or syllable pattern, the child still may be unable to identify them. The way a word or sentence appears in print is not necessarily the way it *sounds* to a hearing-impaired child (for example, the word *money* may be perceived as a one-syllable word). If you have a hearing-loss simulator, use it to listen to the words/sentences from the child's point of view (see Erber 2008). Modify the set of words/sentences to differentiate them further, and then determine if your modification makes auditory identification easier.

After you have written a set of items, you will need to point out the differences in structure and content. This is especially important for a child who relies strongly on sound *patterns*. There are various ways to do this. You can use a colored pen to mark pauses. You can draw lines to describe each pattern: for example, a long line indicates a long sentence; two short lines denote a two-syllable word. Nearly all children quickly learn that line length is analogous to duration. When reading the sentences, you should "act out" the special markings by obscuring your mouth and moving your finger under the sentence as you say the words. When you come to a pause, hold up your hand to indicate "no sound here".

It also is important to describe the *content* of the sentences (i.e., key words and phrases). A simple picture that illustrates the activity, person, or object may be drawn to provide context. Key words should be pointed out both for children who can and cannot read. Some children may be able to read particular syllables or words, but not entire sentences.

The next step is to tell the child that it is time to *listen*. Then obscure your mouth, say one of the items that you have written, and instruct the child to point to and/or repeat the word or sentence as accurately as possible. If the child makes an identification error, use adaptive strategies; for example, repeat the item, articulate more clearly, and/or exaggerate pauses. In some cases, you may decide to decrease the number of response alternatives; for example, cover the top four items, and ask the child to choose from only the bottom two items. A final strategy may be to provide a visible (lipreading) cue. Try several strategies until the child can identify and repeat the spoken item.

You can easily convert this closed-set identification activity into a brief "conversation". After the child has identified a spoken word, phrase, or sentence, ask a comprehension question that is related to that item, and is appropriate to the child's language level. For example, if you presented the word *boots*, and the child identified it correctly, you might ask, "What color are *your* boots?" If the child can answer the related question, reward that response and present another item in the set. If the child cannot answer the question, however, employ various adaptive strategies until the answer is correct (e.g., clarify, simplify the question, provide visible cues).

Using the shared experience approach, you can quickly create a listening activity from anything that happens during the day. This is possible after the child becomes familiar with the procedures, and can anticipate what you will do. When the child sees you write a set of sentences, the child will know it is time to talk about a recent experience and then *listen* as you describe the activity.

Occasionally, you may want to construct sentences for a special purpose. This takes a little more time. See the sentences below: the first set emphasizes *length* difference, and the following three sets are grouped according to *pattern*. These may be used to help a child with poorer listening skills to practice distinguishing sentence lengths and patterns. They also could be used with a child with better listening skills who can recognize constituent words, to provide practice distinguishing between similar sentences within each group.

A set of sentences that differ in length

Mark laughed.
Yvonne likes horses.
Maria wrote a long letter.
Two men will fix the roof today.
After Max cut up the vegetables, he made a salad.
Every morning at 8 o'clock, the family eats breakfast together.

Sets of sentences grouped according to pattern

My teacher bought apples at the shop.
The children played football in the park.
We put our papers on the shelf.
Max saw three elephants at the zoo.

Rrrr! We heard a fire truck on High Street.
Crash! Trudy dropped all the dirty plates.
Hey! You forgot to tie your shoes.
Ouch! I bumped my head on the door.

After playtime, we drank some cold juice.
For breakfast, we ate baked beans and toast.
In this box, there are twelve new pencils.
Under the rock, we found a big lizard.

SPECIFIC LISTENING ACTIVITIES

Specific listening activities can be used to assist in the development of a child's auditory communication skills. For example, you can create special activities for practice on persistent listening difficulties, such as the inability to hear the difference between the words *two* and *three*. Here, the immediate purpose is not to converse fluently through speech, but to concentrate on a specific auditory difficulty. You can use this time to increase your confidence as an instructor and to build the child's confidence as a listener. Select particular listening tasks to satisfy a child's needs as indicated by:

- the results of GASP! (Chapter 4)
- the results of other tests you have administered
- your observations of the child's auditory behavior during daily conversation.

Auditory detection

With appropriate programming/mapping of their personal listening systems, most hearing-impaired children can detect most speech sounds – at least close by in a quiet environment. Regardless, it is important to routinely assess the child's ability to detect the sounds of speech:

- to increase the child's familiarity with the test procedure
- to identify a temporary reduction in hearing sensitivity (e.g., caused by middle-ear disease)
- to verify hearing aids/cochlear implants are working properly
- to determine whether the hearing aids/cochlear implants require reprogramming/re-mapping
- to teach the child to recognize and report a malfunction in the personal listening system
- to identify the basis for any particular difficulties in reception or expression of spoken language (e.g., difficulty distinguishing between *cat* and *cats*)
- to prepare the child for higher-level auditory tasks.

As described in Chapter 4, you can cue an auditory detection task by placing two face pictures (that symbolize sound or no sound) in front of the child (see figure 4.5). With experience, young children will realize that whenever you present those two pictures, you will ask them to indicate whether a sound was audible or not. With older children, the printed words YES and NO alone are sufficient to cue a detection task. Of course, you may allow other responses as well. For example, you may ask the child to place a block in one of two locations, or simply say "yes" or "no" whenever a spoken stimulus is detected or not detected. After repeated practice, you should be able to introduce a detection task when necessary; for example, if you suspect the child's hearing aids are not operating properly, you can quickly check with a speech detection task.

Usually, you will not want to spend much time working at the *detection* level of auditory perception. This procedure is used primarily during an identification or comprehension activity when a child's auditory difficulty seems to be related to an inability to detect a particular item (e.g., the word *two* in "I see two parrots!"). You would then practice detection of that word, changing your voice level, pitch, or sentence context, or pausing before/after the key word to determine the conditions under which the word can be reliably detected.

In addition, you may need to explain and demonstrate that the phoneme /u/ (in the word *two*) is spoken with sound, that the child can detect that vowel under particular conditions (normal voice, near distance, little background noise, functioning listening system), and that the child also must *produce* that vowel with voice – so other people will be able to hear it.

A detection card game

Place a deck of large blank cards on the table. Pick up each one in turn, cover your mouth with the card, speak a phoneme/syllable/word with voice or no voice. Card 1: "/u/" with voice; card 2: "/u/" without voice; card 3: "/u/" without voice; etc. After you present each stimulus, pass the card to the child who must place the card in a YES or NO pile.

Adults should always complete an auditory communication activity with an easy listening task. The aim is to maintain a positive listening attitude. For some children, their most successful listening task will be auditory detection of speech.

Auditory discrimination

The main purpose for an auditory *discrimination* task is to determine why a child exhibits difficulty in identifying a particular spoken item (e.g., the word *take*) and responds with another item instead (e.g., the word *put*). In a discrimination activity, you would speak both words and require the child to indicate whether they sound the same or different. An auditory discrimination task gives the child practice in listening to small differences between spoken items, and helps you understand why a particular auditory misperception has occurred.

A discrimination card game

Place three large blank cards on the table. Pick up each one in turn, cover your mouth with the card, speak a sound/word/phrase, and replace the card in its original position. E.g., Card 1: "mother"; card 2: "mother"; card 3: "brother". Then ask, "Which one is different?" The child must point to the card that was different.

There are several ways to present an auditory discrimination task. For example, you may cover your mouth and say the two words in succession (e.g., "take"…"put"), perhaps gesturing to the right and left as you speak. It is important to gesture in such a way that you establish a "place in space" for each item – the first to your right (child's left) and the second to your left (child's right). Then ask the child if they sound the *same* or *different*. For some children, you may need to ask the question in a more precise manner – "Are they the *same* or *not the same*?" or "Are they the same, *yes* or *no*?" For a young child, it may be necessary to practice first with similar (cup-cup) and dissimilar (cup-toothbrush) objects, each placed in one of two locations.

It is possible to present *more* than *two* spoken units for comparison (Erber 1976; Boothroyd 1991; Hnath-Chisholm et al., 1998). For example, to present three items, cover your mouth and speak each item, again gesturing in such a way as to place each one in a particular location in space. The first item may be "placed" to your right (child's left), the second in front of you (child's center), and the third to your left (child's right). Two of the spoken items should be the same and one different (e.g., /ɑ/-/u/-/ɑ/; dog-dog-cat; in the park-through the park-through the park). Then ask the child "Which is different?" A spoken response is not required – merely pointing to one of three locations is sufficient. This task is a little more difficult than a two-item task because the child must listen for longer and remember more items before responding.

Another approach might be to cover your mouth and produce a sound that changes in quality at random intervals. For example, you may speak a vowel that changes in pitch (ɑ ɑ ɑ ɑ ɑ ɑ ɑ ɑ) or quality (i i i **u** i i i i i), or a word that changes at particular intervals (stop-stop-stop-**top**-stop-stop) (Osberger, Robbins, Miyamoto et al., 1991b; Dawson et al., 1998). The child's task is to indicate when the change occurs, by pointing or saying "now".

Auditory identification

Some hearing-impaired children demonstrate difficulty in identifying particular words or sentences, or in describing their syllable patterns. Others have difficulty understanding instructions or answering questions without visible cues. Both groups may need practice in identifying units of spoken language.

In the first instance, the child needs identification practice to elevate auditory performance to a higher level. In the latter case, the child has demonstrated difficulty at a relatively high level of auditory function, and the adult is interested in discovering the source of the problem; for example, word/sentence length, vocabulary, or language complexity.

The spoken items you ask the child to identify will depend on specific auditory needs. Auditory *identification* practice can be provided with:

- voice pitch (intonation contours)
- vowels, diphthongs

- consonants, consonant blends
- speech sounds in syllable or in word context
- syllables in isolation or in word context
- words in isolation, in phrases, or in sentence context
- phrases in isolation, or in sentence context
- sentences alone, or in the context of narrative
- narrative (stories, songs, rhymes).
  You can establish a limited context for the auditory identification activity by:
- writing a set of items (a list of syllables such as /bi/, /bu/, /pi/, /pu/)
- presenting a small group of objects (*bear, chair, hair, stair*)
- showing pictures that illustrate descriptive sentences (*toy shop, train station, park, supermarket, playground*).

Then name all of the items in the set and tell the child you will say one of the items with your mouth covered. The child needs to listen and indicate which item you spoke by repeating the item or pointing. If the child experiences difficulty, apply common adaptive strategies, that is, repeat, emphasize a syllable or word, clarify your speech, reduce the number of alternatives, and so forth. If the child makes consistent errors, such as confusion between a particular pair of items, present a *discrimination* task with those items.

A simple auditory identification activity involves writing down two speech sounds, words, or phrases that you want the child to compare. Then cover your mouth, point to one of them, and say one of the two items. Ask the child if what you said and what you pointed to are "the same": the child must say "yes" or "no". Items may also be presented in the form of picture cards. In this case, pick up a picture card (e.g., a *blue car*), cover your mouth with the card, either name the picture ("blue car") or say something else ("red bicycle"), then lower the card and ask the child if you named what is shown in the picture – "yes" or "no". Most children enjoy participating in this listening game.

An "easy" auditory identification task might require the child to identify a word from a small set of words with different stress patterns (e.g., *cat, turtle, hot dog, ice-cream cone*). A more difficult listening activity might require the child to identify a word from a set with the same stress pattern (e.g., *dog, leaf, man* or *ice-cream, football, popcorn*) or a set that contains more items (e.g., *fish, house, bird, cup, shoe, pen*). Very difficult listening practice would include words that differ by only one or two vowels or consonants (e.g., *beet, bit, bet* or *spot, pot, pots*).

You can create many listening games that include word or sentence identification (Jennings 1995; Nevins & Chute 1996; Caleffe-Schenck & Baker 2008) (see figure 5.6). Enjoyable listening tasks and appropriate praise/reward can maintain a child's interest and motivation during listening practice. Some children respond well to a positive word, smile, or nod, while others prefer moving a marker along a path to an endpoint, or more tangible reinforcement such as a token. Many children are satisfied to receive the picture cards that depict the spoken items, that is, if the child is correct, the child gets the card; if the child is incorrect, the adult gets the card.

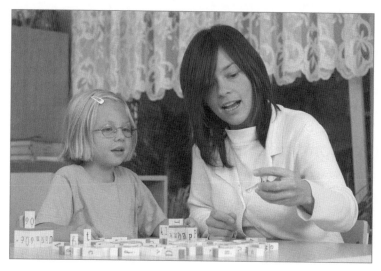

Figure 5.6 **A listening game**

Occasionally, reverse the procedure so that *you* play the role of listener. The *child* presents the phoneme, syllable, or word and *you* indicate when you can or cannot detect, discriminate, or identify the item the child speaks.

A good activity to provide auditory identification practice with phrase- or sentence-length material is called the "Tracking Procedure" (De Filippo & Scott 1978; De Filippo 1988; Goldberg 1988; O'Donoghue et al., 1998). In this procedure, you read a brief story (200 to 500 words) to the child in short "chunks" or "language units" with your mouth obscured. After each language unit is read, the child attempts to repeat what he/she has heard. You choose the length of each language unit (word, phrase, sentence) based on the child's ability and performance. When an identification error occurs, you adapt (repeat, clarify, prompt) until the child can identify what you said. If you need to use gestures or visible articulation to clarify the speech material, mark the locations in the text (e.g., use brackets to indicate natural gestures; use circles to indicate visible cues).

The aim of this activity is to maximize the child's auditory "tracking rate" (in words per minute), while reducing the child's dependence on visual cues. You may obtain the following measures at each practice session to demonstrate progress:

- the tracking rate – i.e., the total number of words in the story divided by the total time required for completion (words per minute)
- the proportion of words presented with visible cues – i.e., the number of words you presented with gestures or visible articulation, divided by the total number of words in the story.

An identification card game

Place a small set of picture cards on the table (e.g., *cow, duck, snail, elephant, kangaroo, butterfly*). Cover your mouth, say one of the words, and ask the child to repeat the word. After the child successfully identifies all the items, play again, but this time whenever the child repeats a word correctly, turn over its picture. When all the pictures have been turned over, play the game again until the child can identify the words although their pictures cannot be seen.

Auditory comprehension

During daily conversation, a child may be able to identify (repeat) a question or request, but not have sufficient confidence to answer or respond. Another child may be able to comprehend and respond to spoken messages confidently, but only when the sentences are short and simple. Each of these children can benefit from listening practice at the *comprehension* level.

A simple comprehension task may involve placing a set of pictures in front of the child to establish a context. For example, you might use pictures of Olympic athletes and talk about various sports. Then you could obscure your mouth and describe each of the pictures:

- The Chinese woman won a gold medal.
- A very tall man jumped over a bar.
- This athlete is throwing a javelin.
- That runner was first in the marathon.

Each time, the child must identify which picture you have described.

Then, with your mouth obscured, ask a question that is related to each picture, for example:

- Who won the silver medal?
- What color is his uniform?
- How long is a javelin?
- What country does he come from?

This time, the child must answer the questions appropriately.

Another comprehension task is to tell a brief story (5 to 10 sentences), ideally one that is familiar and illustrated with colorful pictures. You may choose to tell the story with your mouth obscured (auditory conditions) or visible (auditory-visual conditions). Then ask the child questions about the content while your mouth is not visible:

- Where did Jack go?
- What did he take with him?
- Who did he meet?
- How many beans did he get?

- What kind of beans were they?
- What happened next … ?

Again, the child must answer the questions appropriately.

Many auditory comprehension skills, however, do not fit the simple information-recall format summarized above. Some cognitive tasks that are based on spoken language require a child to listen to details in a question or request, create and manipulate auditory images, and/or remember information received via auditory input.

A simple auditory comprehension activity designed to develop and practice these skills is usually presented without context. The teacher/therapist obscures her mouth and asks brief questions:

- What is the opposite of the word tall? (or dark, rough, etc.)
- Which day comes after yesterday?
- Name a very sweet food.
- What are three sports that you play with a ball?
- What do you think of when I say "bedroom"?
- Are there six legs on my chair?

Some practice questions more likely to appear in real conversations could include (Schery & Peters 2003):

- Who used all the hot water?
- What did you do after school today?
- When does the movie begin?
- Where can I buy some ice-cream?
- Why is the dog barking?

Regardless of the type of question, if the child hesitates, or responds incorrectly, you may repeat, clarify, provide acoustic prompts (e.g.,"not *bathroom*"), or provide visible cues as you speak a key word/phrase (e.g.,"… *after school*").

In a variation on this activity, you may present statements that someone might say in a real conversation, and ask the child to respond appropriately, for example: "If I say this (…), what do you say?"

- I'm tired!
- I don't like cats!
- It's time for dinner.
- My feet hurt!
- This chair isn't very comfortable.
- I want another sandwich.
- Golf is a stupid sport!
- Blue is my favorite color.

The child is expected to: acknowledge ("OK"), agree/disagree ("No, it's not stupid!"), ask a related question ("Why don't you like them?"), or reflect your statement ("Green is *my* favorite color!") (Erber 1996).

During auditory comprehension activities, do not allow the child to repeat your utterance first or wait for you to indicate correct identification, and then respond to your question or assertion. Encourage the child to *listen and think* before responding, in order to establish a natural conversational rhythm, and to increase confidence in listening. If the child exhibits difficulty with this approach, be patient and repeat/clarify if necessary.

Conversation

Conversation is a form of social interaction in which language is used in a reciprocal manner between two (or more) people (Myllyniemi 1986). They exchange ideas, feelings, and opinions according to accepted procedures such as turn-taking and cooperation. People converse for many reasons (e.g., to form/maintain friendships, obtain information, or influence others). Every sustained spoken interaction with a hearing-impaired child is a type of conversation which is likely to depend on successful auditory comprehension. One of the principal aims of listening practice is to prepare the hearing-impaired child for participation in spoken conversations in the world outside the home, clinic, or classroom.

A hearing-impaired child may be able to comprehend spoken sentences when they are presented in isolation, but may struggle to identify, or comprehend the same sentences in the rapid exchange of a conversation. Another child, whose speech reception or expression is not perfect, may have difficulty maintaining the flow ("fluency") of conversation (see pp. 91–2). Each of these children can benefit from conversational experience. A parent, teacher, or therapist can converse with a hearing-impaired child to provide interactive practice in speech reception and expression, and to familiarize the child with the cooperative process of sustained conversation (van Uden 1977).

Simulated conversation – QUEST?AR

You can use many types of practice material to engage a child in conversation. One example is QUEST?AR (Questions for Aural Rehabilitation) (Erber 1984). QUEST?AR is a conversational activity that provides interactive experience with common question-answer sequences (Binnie 1976). The aim of QUEST?AR is to help a child learn to anticipate, comprehend, and respond to familiar spoken question forms.

QUEST?AR can be used to provide practice in auditory or auditory-visual perception of speech. Materials include a half-script framework for conversations, a list of topics, and a sequence of 30 related questions (see below). Each conversational topic is a *place* that you have recently visited (e.g., national park, supermarket, a friend's house, hardware store). The prescribed sequence of questions provides a way for the child to systematically find out about your visit.

QUEST?AR topics and questions (Erber 1984)

Where did you go?

Museum, restaurant, post office, shopping, camping, doctor, zoo, beach, airport, swimming, mountains, picnic, music lesson, Mars, supermarket, and so forth.

Questions:

1. Why did you go there?
2. When did you go?
3. How many people went with you?
4. Who were they?
5. What did you take with you?
6. Where is (the place)?
7. How did you get there?
8. What did you see on the way?
9. What time did you get there?
10. What did you do first?
11. What did you see?
12. How many? What color? etc.
13. What happened at (the place)?
14. What else did you do?
15. What were other people doing at (the place)?
16. What was the most interesting thing you saw?
17. What was the most interesting thing you did?
18. What did you buy?
19. What kind? What flavor? What color? etc.
20. How much did it cost?
21. Did anything unusual happen? What?
22. How long did you stay?
23. What did you do just before you came home?
24. When did you leave?
25. How did you get home?
26. What happened on the way home?
27. What time did you get home?
28. How did you feel then?
29. When are you going back?
30. Do you think I should go sometime? Why?

To use QUEST?AR, give the child the booklet that contains the 30 related questions. The child begins the conversation by asking, "Where did you go?" Select a topic from the list of places, and present this topic to the child unambiguously (e.g., with clear speech, text, or even a photo). The child's task is to ask the full list of questions in sequence, obtaining your answer to each one before proceeding to the next.

If the child cannot understand one of your spoken responses, the child should request appropriate repetition or clarification (see Chapter 7 for further details). "Repair strategies" can often be applied naturally during a QUEST?AR-based conversation if both the adult and the child treat this practice activity as if it were a real conversation, rather than a simulation exercise, for example:

Child: "What did you do first?"

Adult: "We carried the table …"

Child: "You called the *people*?"

Adult: "No. We picked up the table …"
Child: "You picked up the table!"
Adult: "We carried the table …!"
Child: "Oh! You *carried* the table …"
Adult: "Yes, and we put it in the truck …"

Note the beginning and ending times of each QUEST?AR practice session, so you can roughly estimate the child's conversational efficiency, expressed in terms of the number of minutes required to obtain correct answers to all 30 questions. This "score" will improve with the child's increasing experience with question-answer sequences. It may also change according to the familiarity of the *topic* ("place"), and the familiarity and complexity of the *answers* that you provide (e.g., common versus unfamiliar vocabulary; simple versus complex sentences).

It is important to discuss the interactive process with the child after each QUEST?AR session, reviewing conversational sequences that were easy or difficult and also strategies that were effective or inappropriate. An audiovisual recording of the session can help you analyze the child's communicative behavior.

Children report that this interactive activity, in which *they* ask the questions rather than an adult, gives them confidence as communicators (i.e., it is easier), because they can often anticipate the form or content of the answers. Each of the adult's spoken responses is greatly restricted both by the topic (e.g., shopping at a hardware store) and by the nature of each question (e.g., "What time did you get home?"). For example, the response to the child's question: "What time did you get home?" will usually be in the form "6 o'clock", "6:30", or "just after 6". In response to a different question: "How did you get there?", the response is likely to be one of the following: "I walked", "I rode my bicycle", "I drove my car", "I took the bus".

Some children get so interested in these "conversations" they ask related questions that do not even appear in the prescribed QUEST?AR sequence (e.g., "How did the boy get his sock out of the tree?" or "Did you remember to turn off the radio?"). They ask these additional questions because they are interested in the content of the conversation and want to know more about the outcome of your story. Although this question-insertion process will invalidate scoring (timing of sessions), do not discourage a child from asking additional *related* questions. It provides desired practice, and promotes involvement in *real* conversations.

Real conversation

Many simple questions can be used to start *real* conversations with a hearing-impaired child. Some examples include:

• What happened on your birthday?

- Which sports are you good at?
- Where do your cousins live?
- What did you eat for breakfast?
- What makes you happy?
- Do you know a vegetarian?
- Are you good at drawing pictures?
- Have you broken any bones?
- Does your family have a pet?
- Who are your neighbors?
- What will you do this weekend?
- Have you traveled to another country?

If you want to provide practice in natural conversation, but find it difficult to think of something to talk about, a prepared list of potential topics can be useful. See table 5.1 for some examples. You may wish to print these conversational topics, one per card, then shuffle and draw a card at random to obtain a topic.

Table 5.1 **Topics for conversation with children (suggested by children) (Erber 2008)**

pets	picnic	dentist	football	school friends
food	insects	camping	train ride	cricket/softball
books	music	birthday	dinosaurs	songs/singers
parents	clothes	dancing	computers	knitting/sewing
bicycle	fights	teachers	shopping	million dollars
zoo	travel	holidays	tooth fairy	part-time job
garden	doctor	make-up	shoes/boots	three wishes
movies	friends	jewellery	homework	skateboards
toys	school	television	Christmas	brother/sister
beach	Easter	hobbies	my room	collections
cooking	family	weekend	swimming	mobile phone

Measuring conversational fluency

To subjectively assess the quality of a conversation, observe the conversation for two to five minutes. Then use the four-point scale below (see table 5.2) to rate "conversational fluency", that is, the proportion of time the conversation flowed smoothly without long silences or periods of breakdown/repair (Erber 1988, 1996).

Table 5.2 **Conversational fluency rating scale**

Low	1	2	3	4	High

4	Conversation flowed smoothly most of the time
3	Conversation flowed smoothly much of the time
2	Conversation flowed smoothly some of the time
1	Conversation flowed smoothly little of the time

Alternatively, you could use DYALOG conversation-analysis software to measure fluency (see figure 5.7) (Erber 1998). With this method, you must press and hold down the space bar of your computer whenever you observe conversation to be non-fluent as a result of breakdown and repair. This method has several advantages because it:

- is more objective than a rating scale
- evaluates conversational fluency moment-by-moment
- produces a graph and numerical results
- avoids errors that can occur from a subjective rating process.

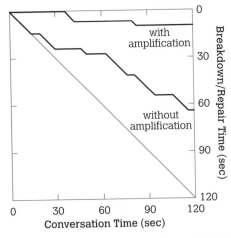

Total: conversation time = two minutes (120 secs)

Conversational breakdown/repair	Without amplif.	With amplif.
Total repair time (sec)	64	8
Per cent of conversation time	53%	7%
Number of repairs	6	2
Average time per repair (sec)	10.7	4.0

Figure 5.7 **Results of conversation analysis with DYALOG software (Erber 2008)**

The results of the subjective method (conversational fluency rating scale) and the objective method (conversation-analysis software) have been found to be correlated (Tye-Murray 2003).

DISCUSSION

The complex process of auditory learning that occurs in each hearing-impaired child is not well understood. The sensations the child receives through hearing aids or cochlear implants are not likely to change as a result of the listening experience. A spoken word's acoustic properties do not change much with repetition. But during the course of days, weeks, or months, the way the brain organizes spoken language and responds to a sound stimulus changes. During bath time, for example, if you say the word "bathtub" to an infant, at first the child may be aware that you have produced sound. After a bit more listening experience, the child may be able to recognize that you have spoken a word containing two syllables. With more listening opportunities, the child may be able to identify the spoken word *bathtub* in context and recognize the object to which it refers. And later, the child may even be able to identify the word without supportive context and comprehend its meaning, although the basic sensation of sound is not much different from before. You have taught the child to analyze, process, and recognize somewhat distorted, ambiguous acoustic cues, and you have given the child confidence to respond appropriately. Very often, auditory development requires simply establishing a listening and learning environment in which the child can succeed and then providing an opportunity for success.

SUMMARY

This chapter has provided a rationale, structure, and direction for a hearing-impaired child's auditory development. There are three general styles of auditory instruction you may apply, each differing in presentation and naturalness: (1) a conversational approach, (2) an experience-based method and (3) practice on specific auditory tasks. With each style, you may apply adaptive procedures in which the child's responses to recent speech-communication activities guide your choice of the next listening task. During this work, you must consider various stimulus types (such as a word or sentence) as well as various response levels (such as identification or comprehension).

It is not necessary for a child's auditory development to follow a prescribed direction or plan where, for example, you present phoneme-detection tasks first and narrative-comprehension last. Instead, you can use a "conversational approach" during all daily interaction, and apply "experience-based" listening practice as a follow-up to each conversation. The adult communicates with the hearing-impaired child in familiar contexts, in approximately the same way as with a child who has normal hearing. If the child fails to comprehend and conversation becomes non-fluent, the adult adapts: repeats/clarifies/simplifies, presents additional (e.g., visible) cues, or requests a lower-level response. The adult applies methods and strategies based on the child's needs at that moment.

As you communicate with the child, you will note consistent errors. Later, you can provide brief periods of specific practice with challenging material. In this way, you can make listening experience a part of all daily interaction, rather than treat listening as a collection of skills to be developed outside the context of everyday communication.

CHAPTER 6

Telephone communication

The most common form of communication through sound *alone* (with no visible cues) is telephone conversation. In recent years, there has been renewed interest in assistive technology and listening methods to make telephone conversation easier for hearing-impaired children.

Telephone conversation is a central part of the daily lives of most people with normal hearing. It plays a major role in business, family, and personal life. Children use the telephone for a variety of reasons, including:

- communication with close relatives
- development and maintenance of social networks
- emergencies – e.g., illness, change of plans, need for transport.

For many hearing-impaired children, however, it may be difficult to converse fluently over a telephone. Communication over a standard telephone is different from face-to-face communication because:

- auditory reception is usually monaural
- the frequency range is limited
- the acoustic output level is limited
- visible cues for communication are not available – e.g., mouth movements, speaker's intent/emotional state, turn-taking.

Various strategies can be used to enhance telephone communication for children with impaired hearing. Some children benefit from accessories and listening devices designed to optimize speech communication over the telephone. They may need specific instruction in using telephone equipment. Other children may need instruction and practice to develop appropriate interactive behavior, auditory communication strategies, and clear speech.

TYPES OF DISTANCE COMMUNICATION

Hearing-impaired children are able to use a variety of different methods for distance communication (Kepler et al., 1992; Harkins & Bakke 2003; Cray et al., 2004; Power & Power 2004; Power et al., 2007). These methods include:

- text communication over the telephone
- text communication over the internet
- audiovisual communication over the internet
- telephone relay service, speech-to-text – i.e., the child talks > the communication partner listens and talks > an intermediary listens and types the partner's message > the child reads the relayed message
- simplified voice communication over the telephone: the child speaks > the communication partner uses a small set of responses or sends messages coded as intensity patterns
- speech communication over the telephone – i.e., the child uses a telephone and ordinary spoken messages for both reception and expression.

We will be concerned mainly with the last method, which relies on hearing and speech for communication over the telephone.

TELEPHONE LISTENING AIDS AND LISTENING METHODS

Hearing-impaired children differ in their auditory skills and so they use different types of personal listening systems. Consequently, they receive auditory input from a telephone in many ways (Compton 2000; Crandell & Smaldino 2002; Bankaitis 2008). In general, only children with mild hearing losses will be able to use a telephone without any type of supplementary amplification. Some children with a moderate hearing loss may simply hold the telephone beside the microphone of their amplification system. Others prefer to use a supplementary amplification system, which usually has the advantage of avoiding feedback squeal and enabling better speech perception.

Different types of supplementary listening apparatus are available for telephone communication. The devices include:

- a telephone amplifier to increase the output level of the telephone by up to 20 dB – built-in type, portable type, replacement handset, in-line external amplifier
- a speakerphone to provide an acoustic link to the microphone of the child's personal listening device

- a soft plastic enclosure ("coupler") to improve delivery of sound from the telephone to a hearing aid microphone
- an electro-magnetic "telecoil" or "loop" to receive electromagnetic signals from some telephones
- a direct (electrical or wireless) connection between the telephone and the hearing aid or cochlear implant, which bypasses the earphone of the telephone and the microphone of the personal listening device.

Children with similar hearing may differ in their preferences for supplementary listening apparatus. This could be due to:

- differences in magnetic field strength produced by different telephones
- differences in the sensitivity of their hearing aid telecoils
- differences in gain or frequency response between the "T" (telephone) and "M" (microphone) settings of a given hearing aid (Thompson 2002)
- cumulative distortions that can occur when several electrical/digital devices are used together to convey sound from the telephone to the ear – e.g., a supplementary amplifier and a hearing aid/cochlear implant
- differences in voice pitch, intensity, and speech quality of communication partners.

To achieve the best speech communication over a telephone system, the child must have the opportunity to experiment with a variety of supplementary listening devices and select one that provides the greatest intelligibility when conversing with regular communication partners.

PROCEDURES FOR USING TELEPHONE EQUIPMENT

To use a telephone effectively, a child must first learn how to recognize common telephone sounds, and learn the procedures for using different types of telephone apparatus.

Preliminary procedures

A young child may need to learn several methods for activating a telephone. These could include:

- lifting the handset from its cradle – e.g., home phone
- pressing the "on" button – e.g., mobile phone
- inserting coins or a phone card – e.g., public phone
- dialing 0 for an outside line – e.g., business phone.

Telephone sounds

The child will need to learn to detect and recognize common telephone sounds such as:

- steady dial tone – the child must wait to hear the dial tone, which indicates the system is ready to accept a dialed number
- incoming call: telephone ringing – the child must be able to recognize the ringing of an incoming call in ambient noise. There are many alternative ring tones, and they differ in audibility
- outgoing call: phone ringing – a repeating sound pattern which indicates the dialed phone is ringing
- silence – may indicate the dialed number is incomplete or incorrect, the phone battery is low, a fault exists in the phone system, etc.
- recorded message – e.g., answering machine/voice mail, a spoken/button-press response is required, the dialed phone is out of service, the number has been changed
- engaged/busy signal – indicates a conversation is in progress, try again later
- voice says "hello" – someone is ready to converse (which may be the desired person or someone else).

Obtaining a connection

The child may need to learn how to obtain a connection in different ways such as:

- pressing the numeral keypad in the desired sequence and then pressing "enter"
- finding a stored number in the phone memory and then selecting it
- searching a personal directory and selecting the correct number.

Beginning and ending procedures

Each step of a telephone conversation is guided by socially accepted procedures (Hopper 1992). Some "rules" for interaction are unique to telephone conversation (e.g., opening and closing rituals), and some vary between cultures (e.g., greetings). Both participants in a telephone conversation usually have goals. One function of a conversation is to coordinate the discourse to reach these goals.

To start any conversation, a person must obtain and hold the communication partner's attention, and the communication partner must show willingness to participate. In a telephone conversation, the ring of the telephone (initiated by the caller) gets the partner's attention. When the partner answers the telephone and says "Hello!" this indicates that person's willingness to converse. The greeting signals the caller to continue and to introduce a topic. Socially accepted procedures require the person who answers the telephone to speak first.

Typically, the *caller* is expected to manage the first part of the conversation. If the caller is a hearing-impaired child whose speech quality is unusual, this can momentarily confuse the person receiving the call. To minimize difficulty, the conversation can begin slowly to give the other person an opportunity to orient perceptually to the child's speech. The child could be encouraged to say, "I have a hearing problem, so please talk slowly and carefully. I will talk carefully too. Then we can both understand."

To end a conversation smoothly, the two communicators must follow a socially accepted pattern. There are two main steps: first, they agree to end the conversation; and second, they actually end it (Schegloff & Sacks 1973). Usually the caller suggests that the conversation might end, and the other person typically accepts this suggestion. The caller might say "I've got to go now" and the other person might say "OK". The caller then says, "Good-bye", the other person replies similarly, and the conversation ends. Most telephone conversations tend to end slowly, rather than abruptly.

Young children generally learn attention-getting and turn-taking procedures relatively easily, but take much longer to acquire the appropriate forms of opening and closing rituals.

Turn-taking behavior

Both telephone communicators must agree on an orderly method of talking. Conversational experience is required to fill silences or to help the other person during the turn-taking process, because neither can see the other, and important visual cues such as eye contact, gestures, posture, and expression are not available. Some general rules are that:

- each person must have a regular turn to talk
- only one person may talk at a time
- silences between utterances must be brief.

The messages exchanged during a conversational turn-taking sequence usually form a closely related "contingent pair". There are various types of contingent pairs, including:

Greeting: "Hello! Martin speaking."
Greeting: "Hi, this is Anne."
Question: "Is Auntie Sue there?"
Answer: "Yeah ..... I'll get her."
Request: "Auntie Sue ... Can you come to my birthday party?"
Acceptance: "Yes, I'd love to ... On Saturday? ... What time?"
Offer: "Should I wear my fairy wings?"
Rejection: "Oh no! Please don't, Auntie Sue!"

Assertion:	"My mum is going to make cupcakes!"
Question:	"With pink icing?"
End (suggestion):	"Well, I've got to go now!"
End (agreement):	"OK, I'll see you on Saturday!"
End (final):	"Bye!"
End (final):	"Bye!"

These two-part contingent pairs contribute to conversation in several ways. The second part is not only a response to the first part but also signals that the respondent is willing to cooperate at that point in the conversation – and invites the other person to continue. Turn-taking routines allow a child to begin a conversation, make plans, give/get information, change topics, and end the conversation. Most conversations are coordinated through spoken patterns learned from participation and experience. For more examples of contingent pairs, (see pp. 122–3).

EVALUATING TELEPHONE COMMUNICATION ABILITY

The first step in helping a child to become a successful telephone communicator is to evaluate the child's motivation, experience, listening preferences, and auditory skills. The findings will suggest appropriate goals and procedures.

Ask

Ask the child about his/her personal motivation, experience and preferences with telephone communication. This could include:

- why the child wants to use the telephone
- how the child prefers to listen during a telephone conversation (e.g., external amplifier, telecoil, direct audio input, etc.)
- whether the child feels that some people are easier to understand than others. Who? Why?
- whether some conversational topics are preferred or avoided.

Observe

Observe behavior as another person engages the child in simple telephone conversations on familiar topics – e.g., pets, holidays, or favorite sports. Note the following:

- the child's ability to understand by listening alone
- how the child begins and ends a conversation
- turn-taking behavior

- avoidance of interruptions and long silences
- the child's own speech intelligibility
- self-clarification of speech misunderstood by others
- confidence as an auditory communicator
- apparent level of anxiety and stress
- reliance on the partner's patience and cooperation
- the person who manages the conversation – is it the child or the communication partner?
- appropriate use of clarification requests
- reliance on particular clarification-request strategies.

Assess

Child's listening skills

A list of simple questions can help you estimate how well a child is able to hear and respond appropriately over the telephone (Plant et al., 1980):

- What is your last name?
- How old are you?
- When were you born?
- What is your father's first name?
- How many brothers and sisters do you have?
- What is the name of your street?
- Do you live in a house or an apartment?
- What is your telephone number?
- What is your favorite color?
- Which television program do you like the best?

Child's speech intelligibility

It is important to evaluate the child's speech early in a telephone instruction program, to identify any potential obstacles to conversational fluency. Determine whether just a few speech sounds are produced imprecisely, or whether the child has more significant disorders of articulation, timing, and prosody. If intelligibility is low, telephone communication will be disrupted repeatedly by requests for clarification from the communication partner.

When assessing speech, it is important to exclude visible cues, so intelligibility through a telephone is not overestimated (Monsen 1983a). Audio samples of speech may be recorded as the child produces a list of sentences. Intelligibility can be scored in terms of key words identified correctly (McGarr 1983; Boothroyd 1984), or rated on a scale from unintelligible to intelligible (Allen et al., 1998; O'Donoghue et al., 1999). The child's speech intelligibility is likely to vary as a function of the listener's familiarity and experience (e.g., the child's mother is likely to understand more than a stranger).

The child's use of adaptive strategies as a speaker also may be assessed (Lloyd 1999). Is the child aware of his/her own acoustic speech intelligibility? Can the child clarify his/her own speech when communicating? Are self-clarification strategies appropriate and effective?

RESULTS OF ASSESSMENT

Most hearing-impaired children can be placed into one of three general categories of telephone-communication ability:

- Group 1 can communicate fluently over the telephone with few auditory errors and little need for repetition/clarification by the communication partner.
- Group 2 can communicate adequately over the telephone with a familiar person who knows the child's vocabulary and language level, and who repeats, clarifies, and provides context when necessary.
- Group 3 can identify only simple spoken messages over the telephone, or may rely on an acoustic intensity pattern code. Their auditory word-identification ability over the telephone is poor.

FACTORS THAT AFFECT EASE OF TELEPHONE COMMUNICATION

Three factors need to be considered at all times during telephone communication practice. These factors influence the difficulty of each practice activity.

WHO IS THE COMMUNICATION PARTNER?

This could be a family member, experienced therapist/teacher, close friend, cooperative person, or unhelpful stranger.

HOW ACCESSIBLE IS THE COMMUNICATION PARTNER?

Accessibility can vary from face-to-face with no barrier, face-to-face with a barrier, a nearby room, or remote/distant communication.

WHAT IS THE NATURE OF THE CONVERSATION?

This may be a script, half-script, specific practice activity, role-play, or unlimited conversation.

Figure 6.1 can be used to illustrate the relationship between these factors. The easiest communication condition (A) for most hearing-impaired children is one in which the communication partner is familiar and cooperative (e.g., a parent, teacher, or therapist); this person is easily accessible (e.g., in the same room); and the conversation is pre-arranged (e.g., a printed script). The most difficult condition (Z) is one in which the partner is a stranger with no experience communicating with a hearing-impaired child (e.g., a man at a bicycle shop); is not accessible (e.g., two kilometres distance); and the content of the conversation is not anticipated (e.g., "Hi! This is Jason at *Mike's Bikes.* We fixed your front tire. You can pick up your bike this afternoon") (Anderson et al., 2006). Intermediate conditions of difficulty exist between these extremes. The adult's role is to help the child advance along each dimension.

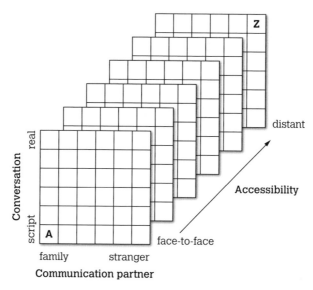

Figure 6.1 **Factors that affect the ease of telephone communication for a hearing-impaired child (adapted from Erber 1985)**

TELEPHONE COMMUNICATION PRACTICE

Telephone-communication practice can incorporate a variety of activities, depending on the child's listening and speech skills, spoken language, and experience communicating without visible cues over a telephone.

Closed-circuit telephone system

Many activities can be facilitated by using a system that permits flexibility in the location of the adult and the child.

General configurations include (see figure 6.2):

a   The adult and the child sit in the same room. The therapist obscures her mouth but may provide visible cues when the child needs clarification, prompting, or another form of assistance. This near condition is used to familiarize the child with basic telephone-communication procedures.

b   The adult and the child sit in nearby rooms without visual contact. They participate in simple telephone conversations. This intermediate condition helps the child develop independence and confidence. The adult is accessible if help is required.

c   The adult and the child sit in distant rooms. The therapist is not accessible. The child must be self-reliant throughout the conversation, getting/giving information and requesting/providing clarification.

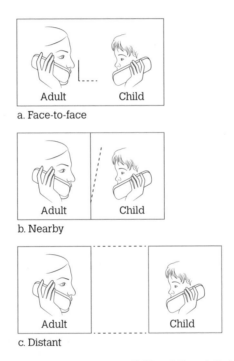

Figure 6.2 **How to vary accessibility of the adult during telephone communication practice (adapted from Erber 1985)**

These degrees of accessibility range from closely supervised communication to independent communication. Not all children progress quickly through all three levels. Some lack the listening skills and confidence to communicate fluently without visible cues. The adult's role is to facilitate auditory communication potential. This may be achieved by employing a progressive approach in which accessibility is gradually reduced, and increased independence is encouraged.

Pre-recorded messages

Some hearing-impaired children want to communicate over the telephone for social reasons, but they are anxious about conversing with a person who is not visibly present. To obtain auditory experience without interacting with an actual communication partner, a child may practice listening to *pre-recorded* messages.

The adult can give the child a list of numbers to dial, which access pre-recorded commercial messages about products/services, opening times, airline schedules, and so forth. The child listens through a telephone and personal listening system. This activity is motivating and relatively stress-free, but some children complain that recorded speakers present their information too quickly and/or without clarity. Poor recording quality, a weak speech signal, audio distortion, and/or background noise can also make listening difficult.

> ### Content of a pre-recorded commercial message
> [Fitzroy Veterinary Clinic: 9489-2195]
> "The Fitzroy Veterinary Clinic is currently closed. Our opening hours are 8 AM to 8 PM Monday through Friday, 9 AM to 4 PM on Saturday, and 10 AM to 2 PM on Sunday. If you have an after-hours emergency, please call the Animal Accident and Emergency Center on 9379-0700. Thank you for your call."

An adult can supplement pre-recorded commercial messages with other recorded messages relevant to the child. An example is "school news" containing the daily menu, after-school activities, or general information. The structure and content can be modeled on commercial pre-recorded messages, but the school messages can be simplified with regard to vocabulary, language, and length. The speaker should be instructed to speak slowly and carefully.

> ### "School News" for listening practice
> "Today's lunch special is sausage pizza."
> "The band will practice after school today in the music room between 3:30 and 5:00 PM."
> "Please park your bicycles at the school sports center and not by the front entrance."
> "Tomorrow's weather will be cloudy in the morning, with rain in the afternoon. The temperature will be 16°C."

A set of comprehension questions can be used to focus the child's attention and establish a purpose for this listening activity. Comprehension questions could be in the format "When is the veterinary clinic open on Sunday?" or "What is today's lunch special?" A fill-in-the-blank format could also be used, in which parts of spoken sentences appear as text, and other parts as blank spaces. Ask the child to listen and supply the missing information. To make this task easier, you may list three or four alternative responses to choose from. As the child's confidence increases, you can withdraw print alternatives and present the listening task in an open-set format.

The tracking procedure

The tracking procedure (De Filippo & Scott 1978; De Filippo 1988, see p. 85) is an *identification* task that can be used to provide listening practice over the telephone. In this procedure, the adult reads parts of a story or article. The child listens and attempts to repeat word-for-word what was said. The adult speaks the material in segments. The length (sentences, phrases, words) depends on the ease with which the child receives the spoken messages. Although the adult usually selects communication strategies when difficulty occurs, the child may request a preferred method of clarification. The adult may need to repeat, exaggerate, increase voice level, simplify, or provide synonyms (Erber & Greer 1973; Tye-Murray 1994; Erber 1996).

This task usually requires an orientation session. During this session, the adult and the child must agree on spelling code words for letters of the alphabet (e.g., a = Afghanistan; b = basketball; c = caterpillar; etc.) and short phrases for cueing the use of particular strategies (e.g., "say it again" to indicate repetition or "different sentence" to indicate placement of a difficult word in another context).

To avoid long delays and confusion, simply bypass spoken items that the child cannot identify after three repetitions/clarifications. Make a list of these items for later discussion. The difficulty of particular words or phrases will depend on the child's hearing loss, personal listening system, telephone-coupling device, listening experience, vocabulary, language level, and many other factors.

The tracking rate achieved is the number of words in the story or article divided by the number of minutes required to complete the task. The results of several telephone-tracking sessions are shown in figure 6.3. The participants were two severely hearing-impaired 18-year-old males who were regular hearing aid users. They could engage in simple telephone conversations with family and close friends but needed practice in spoken interaction with strangers. Both teenagers increased their auditory tracking rate while communicating with a therapist. Their words-per-minute rate after six to seven sessions, however, was still below the rate they could achieve through face-to-face communication while listening through their hearing aids.

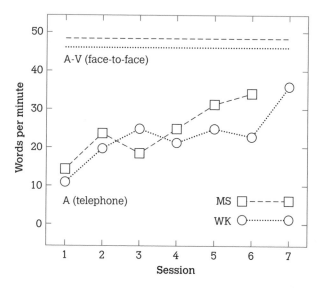

Figure 6.3 **Results of telephone tracking (adapted from Erber 1982)**

Telephone scripts

Scripted activities are ideal for orienting a child to the turn-taking patterns of simple conversation. They help the child become familiar with various types, contents, and functions of telephone conversation; for example, get help, social interaction, obtain information, make plans.

FULL SCRIPT

In this activity, the dialog is written in advance. The adult and the child each receive a copy of the script, and they take turns reading/speaking their parts. A full script eliminates most of the anxiety and stress that can result from a real conversation.

HALF SCRIPT

In this activity, the child receives a printed list of questions, and asks these in sequence. The adult responds and the child listens. For each question, the response set may be open (any response is possible) or may be artificially limited (the child chooses from a small set of possible responses: *soup, salad, sushi, sandwich*).

QUEST?AR (Erber 1984, 1996) is a half-script communication activity that can be used to simulate a telephone conversation. The booklet contains 30 questions in a prescribed sequence that can refer to a variety of topics selected from a list. The child asks each question and must obtain the adult's answer before proceeding to the next question. If the adult cannot understand the content of a question spoken by the child, or the child cannot understand the adult's spoken answer, both must apply strategies to achieve intelligibility before they can proceed with the conversation. Administration of QUEST?AR is described in Chapter 5 (see pp. 88–90).

In a variation of the QUEST?AR activity, the child is given the name of a cooperative adult (e.g., a student teacher), the adult's telephone number, and a set of questions that establish a framework for a brief telephone conversation. The child's task is to obtain answers to the questions. The adult is given a list of clarification strategies the child is likely to request (see p. 112) and a brief explanation of how to help the child maintain the flow of conversation. This type of interactive listening activity can be used with children who have adequate auditory skills and sufficient confidence to engage in a telephone conversation with an unfamiliar person.

Questions for a brief conversation

Where were you born?
Where do you live now?
What did you like to do when you were a teenager?
Where did you go to school?
What were your favorite subjects?
Which is your favorite football/soccer/hockey team?
What kind of food do you like to cook/eat?
What are your hobbies?
What kind of movies do you like?
What will you do this weekend?

Listening games

In a typical "referential communication" listening game, one person (usually an adult) speaks instructions, directions, or information without visible cues to another person (usually a child) across a barrier (Greenspan et al., 1975; Yule 1997; Lloyd et al., 2005; also (see pp. 71–2). This type of listening game can be easily adapted to telephone communication practice (Lloyd 1991, 1992).

Example 1: Who/what am I?

This activity enables the child to learn how to obtain information by asking questions. The adult writes the name of a person, animal, place, or object, and may provide a clue: I work in this building, I live on a farm, I am a famous monument, I am in the playground. The child tries to discover the identity by asking questions: Are you a teacher? What do you eat? Are you in France? Are you metal? This procedure may also be reversed to give the child practice in listening and *answering* questions.

Example 2: News reporter

In this activity the child asks a sequence of questions to find out about an event or experience that happened to the communication partner. The adult has witnessed an auto accident, watched a sporting event, met a famous person, etc. The child plays the role of a news reporter and must find out what happened by asking relevant questions: "What happened first?" "What did the policeman do?" "What was the final score?" "What was she wearing?"

Example 3: Where did I go?

This activity requires the child to ask questions to find out about the adult's experiences (similar to QUEST?AR, but *without* a half-script). The adult names a place visited and the child tries to find out more details: "Did you take the bus?" "When did the store open?" "Where did you eat lunch?" "What did the parrot say?"

Example 4: Here, there, everywhere

This activity gives the child structured experience in following map directions (Lloyd 1991, 1992). The adult describes a route from home or school to a destination such as a bus stop, train station, or shopping center: "Walk through the park to Wellington Road, turn left and go two blocks, turn right at Hastings Street." The child traces the route on a map and, if necessary, may ask confirming questions such as "Turn right at *Station* Street?"

Example 5: Picture

In this activity the child learns how to provide an accurate description by drawing a picture and describing the picture to the adult, who attempts to draw a similar picture according to the description. The adult may or may not show the child the picture after each step. The child and adult compare their pictures on completion and discuss sources of error.

Example 6: Bingo!

This activity helps the child learn to identify words, phrases, and sentences commonly used in telephone conversation. The adult writes items in the squares of a large Bingo card: Is your mother home? Who's speaking? Hello! Good-bye! The adult then speaks these items randomly. The child listens to each item and places a marker in the corresponding square. When all squares are marked, the child says "Bingo". The child and adult then discuss any errors.

Example 7: People and places

This activity gives the child experience in obtaining detailed information and requesting clarification. The adult prepares a list of names, addresses, and telephone numbers (e.g., Bala Lingam; 195 Whitehorse Road; 9878-1597). The adult then speaks and clarifies each item for the child as requested, who attempts to obtain all the information correctly through careful listening, requesting specific clarification (e.g., "Please say the name very slowly"), and confirming details (e.g., "Did you say 199?").

Role-play

Role-play activities serve as a transition to actual, unstructured conversations. No script or half script is provided. Instead, each participant (adult and child) plays a role in a specified situation. The child is given a communication task; for example, obtain information from a friend, deliver a birthday greeting to a grandparent, receive a message for another family member, request help in an emergency, plan to meet at a particular time and place, or order a pizza. The adult plays the corresponding role.

Real conversation

The child and a communication partner converse for two to five minutes on a topic selected from a list (see table 5.1). The adult rates conversational fluency on a four-point scale (see table 5.2). The child's progress is assessed weekly.

Intensity pattern codes

The use of intensity pattern codes for telephone communication is mostly helpful for children with profound hearing losses who can identify only the intensity patterns of spoken messages (McLeod & Guenther 1977; Castle 1978; Erber 1985). This method was more commonly used prior to the advent of cochlear implants, mobile phones, and text messages. One of the simplest applications of this method requires the hearing-impaired child to converse by asking yes/no questions. The normal-hearing communication partner responds by saying "yes-yes" (two syllables), or "no" (one syllable). The procedure is especially valuable in emergencies where other means of communication are not available.

REPAIRING COMMUNICATION BREAKDOWN

Communication breakdown can occur when a hearing-impaired child converses over the telephone. Potential sources of breakdown include:
- a communication partner speaking too quickly and without clarity
- a communication partner being impatient or uncooperative
- introduction of new topics without warning.

When communication breaks down and becomes non-fluent, an appropriate strategy must be used to restore the flow of conversation (Castle 1988). There are two main steps:

1 identify the source of difficulty
2 overcome the difficulty.

Avoidance and/or resolution of difficulty may require the child to:
- recognize and acknowledge confusion/misunderstanding
- check the personal listening system and accessory device
- test and replace batteries
- find a quieter place
- guide the partner through resolution of the difficulty
- ask the partner to speak slowly and clearly
- ask the partner to clarify (e.g., repeat, use synonyms or re-phrase sentences)
- clarify own speech and/or language.

Some strategies may also be used pre-emptively to prevent breakdown before it occurs (e.g., finding a quiet place to talk). You can help the child prepare for these events by simulating difficulties and enacting repair scenarios (see Chapter 7 for more information about conversation management and repair strategies).

Communication partners can use a variety of clear speech and language strategies to avoid or resolve communication breakdown (Erber 1985, 1996; Tye-Murray & Schum 1994; see also Chapter 9). These strategies include:
- reducing background noise
- speaking with adequate voice level
- speaking slowly and carefully
- pausing between syllables/words
- avoiding rare words
- using simple syntax
- spelling words (although this approach can introduce difficulties of its own if the child confuses the letter names (e.g., c-t-p or f-s-x)
- using spelling code words (e.g., a = Afghanistan) – this can be an effective but time-consuming process.

Resolution is usually quicker and easier if the *child* can accurately judge the reason for the communication breakdown and then guide the partner to modify speech and/or language to repair the breakdown. A child who knows how to request clarification in specific ways can usually sustain a telephone conversation. Rather than simply asking, "What?" for example (which will probably elicit a repetition response), the child might ask, "Are you still talking about your new shoes?" (to verify the topic) (see Chapter 7 for more detail).

Communication difficulties and clarification requests	
Speech too fast >	"Please speak slower."
Speech too soft >	"Please speak a little louder."
Speech unclear >	"Could you please say that another way?"
Sentence too long >	"Please say that in a shorter sentence."
Unsure of topic >	"Are you still talking about … "
Background noise >	"I hear noise. Please go to a quiet place."
Listening system >	"Excuse me a minute. I need to check my hearing aids/ cochlear implant."

ORGANIZATION OF PRACTICE SESSIONS

A typical telephone-communication practice session may include:

1 informal discussion of previously successful strategies
2 a brief orientation to the planned practice activity
3 communication practice (e.g., question-answer, auditory "tracking", brief conversation). The degree of partner accessibility can be varied as per figure 6.2
4 review of persistent auditory communication difficulties (e.g., inability to distinguish /m, n/), and the relative benefits of particular clarification strategies to resolve these difficulties.

MEASURING PROGRESS

A child's progress as a telephone communicator can be measured by sampling the child's performance on a variety of listening tasks. The "Pediatric Telephone Profile" (Tait et al., 2001) is a rating scale that includes skills ranging from simple ("detects ringing sound of telephone") to complex ("participates in open conversation with an unfamiliar speaker") (see figure 6.1 and Pediatric Telephone Profile points below). A child's performance on each task is scored as "never" (0), "sometimes" (1), or "always" (2). A child's score will typically reflect the amount of telephone-communication experience.

Pediatric Telephone Profile (Tait et al., 2001)

- detects ringing sound of telephone
- identifies ringing sound
- detects dial tone
- identifies dial tone
- detects voice
- identifies a known speaker
- identifies the word "Hello!"
- identifies the word "Bye-bye!"
- identifies own name
- identifies names of colors (from a set of four)
- identifies names of family members
- identifies days of the week
- identifies numbers (from 1 to 10)
- follows structured conversation from a script
- follows structured conversation without a script
- participates in open conversation with a familiar speaker
- participates in open conversation with an unfamiliar speaker

SUMMARY

Hearing-impaired children differ in their ability to communicate over the telephone. Factors that affect this ability include:

- adequacy of the equipment that is used
- the child's experience with telephone-communication procedures
- the amount of specific instruction received
- the child's listening skills
- the child's general knowledge of spoken language
- the child's ability to apply clarification strategies
- intelligibility of the child's own speech
- patience and cooperation from communication partners.

Many special auditory activities are available for listening practice: attention to details in recorded messages; repetition of narrative ("tracking"); participation in simulated conversations; role-play; and use of spelling or pattern codes devised specifically for telephone communication. The role of the parent or teacher is to eliminate as many obstacles as possible to help the hearing-impaired child reach his/her potential for telephone communication. A progressive approach to communicative independence may be employed, in which the adult gradually increases distance and decreases accessibility.

CHAPTER 7

[*Conversation management*

In previous chapters, we have described ways to help a hearing-impaired child develop auditory communication skills. In this chapter, we will discuss strategies that can be used to increase the child's understanding of what people say, and to maintain the fluency of conversation.

CAUSES AND EFFECTS OF MISPERCEPTION

Hearing-impaired children will often misperceive parts of conversations in which they participate. These misunderstandings can be caused by various factors (Lloyd 1999) including:

- the child's hearing impairment
- the communication partner's lack of clarity
- complexity of spoken language
- unfamiliar vocabulary
- topic shifts
- incomplete input: acoustic cues only – the person's mouth was not visible (e.g., over the telephone, or if the person turned around)
- incomplete input: visible cues only (e.g., the person was too far away, or the voice level was too soft; the listening system was not working properly, or the battery was low)
- the communication partner's message was neither heard nor seen (e.g., the child was not paying attention)
- environmental distractions.

A spoken message may be misperceived in different ways as shown below. For example, during a conversation, a child may confidently hear her mother say, "Next Friday, we'll eat dinner at grandma's house." If this spoken message answers a question, or logically follows her mother's previous sentence, the child can assume she understood what her mother said.

A hearing-impaired child may misperceive a spoken message in different ways

Meaningful but incorrect – the message seems to fit the conversation, but perception was incorrect. For example, while cooking with onions: *"They baked a pie."* Actually spoken: "They'll make you cry."

Meaningless message with confidence – the message appears to be perceived clearly, but doesn't make sense or fit the conversation. For example, "What did he say?" *"He wants a furry apple."* Actually spoken: "He wasn't very helpful."

Nonsense – a series of meaningless syllables is perceived. For example, "Did you finish your homework?" *"Mau fitr pekd laimmi aruipeng!"*

Fragments – only part of the message is received, perhaps incorrectly. For example, "Why didn't you buy the chair?" – *"Because we saw … in the shop window."*

Later, however, the child may hear her uncle say something that doesn't seem to make sense in the framework of the conversation: "The walrus was thinking …". The child may suspect she has misunderstood and may ask her uncle for help: "Did you say … the walrus?" At another time, the child could be *certain* that she misunderstood what her aunt said, because most of it was not intelligible: "I'll kaepoo sottum ung appletake". In this case, the child and her aunt must work together to increase the intelligibility of the aunt's message. This may involve modifying the content of the message and/or the way it was spoken.

CONTEXT AND INTELLIGIBILITY

Upon receiving an unclear spoken message, a child may unconsciously employ linguistic and cognitive processes to identify what the communication partner said. If the topic is familiar, and the child can recall the recent flow and content of the conversation, the child may be able to "guess" the nature of the unclear message. The child may rely on recent memory to recall what preceded the spoken sentence, or apply word associations and basic rules of word order to reconstruct the spoken message. This approach to recovery and identification of an unclear message is an example of "top-down" language processing, which is a high-level metalinguistic skill (Lubinsky 1986; Chermak & Musieck 2002; MacIver-Lux, 2009). While some children are able to do this without conscious effort, others may need specific practice to help them learn these skills.

When an audiologist presents words or sentences as test items in the clinic, they are usually unrelated and presented in an arbitrary sequence. In real life, however, people usually speak in a meaningful *context*, that is, in a situation that includes the communicators and their surroundings, a topic, an activity, and related words/ sentences. In many cases, the situation itself may prompt or stimulate a person to say something. Conversational context can provide clues to what the person has just said, is now saying, or is likely to say next. Some situations are so closely associated with particular messages, in fact, that a child often can *anticipate* what an adult will say. For example, a parent holding two pieces of fruit might say: "Would you like an apple or a banana for lunch?"

A hearing-impaired child who is aware of the conversational context (and how it can affect what someone might say) is much more likely to identify an ambiguous message than a child who relies exclusively on acoustic speech information. Parents and teachers have observed that a child who makes use of contextual information will usually receive more of the message correctly when it is first spoken, will require fewer repetitions and clarifications, and will experience greater fluency in conversation.

Several types of context can contribute to conversational fluency including:

- location and situation
- word order
- interpersonal context
- word/phrase relationships
- conversational sequences.

Location and situation

A conversation always takes place *somewhere*, and usually between two or more people who are doing *something*. The particular situation that prompted the conversation and the surroundings where it occurs often influence what the communicators say to one another. For example, if the conversation occurs in a restaurant, at least some of the conversation will concern the topics of food and drink. In addition, within the restaurant environment, even the immediate situation may affect the flow of the conversation; for example, "I dropped my fork!" or "I love this spaghetti!"

Daily situations establish a context for conversation and can help a child anticipate spoken messages. We often expect people to express themselves in ways that are appropriate to their roles. For example, if a boy scout arrives at your door with a box of chocolate bars, he can be expected to say something like: "Hello. We're selling chocolate to raise money ...". With a little practice, a child can learn to use similar contextual prompts to anticipate what people might say. Several assessment and practice procedures have been based on this principle (Morkovin 1947; Jeffers & Barley 1971; Garstecki & O'Neill 1980; Chermak 1981; Kaplan et al., 1987) (see examples of context below).

> **Context affects what people say**
>
> **A. Messages spoken in particular *situations***
> At a jewellery shop: "Everything is so expensive!"
> Waiting for a train: "The train is late again!"
> At a restaurant: "This menu is in *French!*"
>
> **B. Messages spoken by particular *people***
> Mother: "Go and ask your father!"
> Sister: "Did you borrow my red belt?"
> Teacher: "You have two weeks to finish this assignment!"

Interpersonal context

The relationship between the communicators also establishes a context. In this interpersonal space, only particular topics are likely to be discussed and certain levels of discourse reached (Watzlawick et al., 1967). If the communicators share many experiences, feelings, or opinions, it is likely they will interact within this familiar framework. If a child knows what the other person is likely to *think* or *feel* in a particular situation, this is a clue to what that person might say in that situation.

Even if the communicators have just met and are unfamiliar with one another, people quickly form impressions based on a new awareness of the other's personality and interests. These suppositions regarding the other person, if correct, can guide a hearing-impaired child to accurately anticipate the content of spoken messages and style of interaction (Clark & Clark 1977). Moreover, while speaking, a person may produce non-verbal prompts or clues to the meaning of an utterance, such as facial expression, eye contact, posture, or gestures (Berger & Popelka 1971; Argyle 1988).

Word/phrase relationships

We use *words* to communicate, and we employ words in sequences (i.e., phrases and sentences) to communicate efficiently. The grammar of our language specifies the order in which we must speak words to convey our intended meaning. These formal rules of word order produce a degree of redundancy and predictability within sentences. For example, given the sentence fragment, "The carpenter hammered a ... " we reasonably presume that this sequence of words will end with a noun, or perhaps an adjective-noun pair. This predictability can often enable a child to resolve a misunderstanding. A child with knowledge of spoken language can use linguistic context to recover unclear messages (Alyeshmerni & Taubr 1975).

Some words are so closely associated with others that they regularly occur in the same sentence. Some connections between words are very strong, as the result of word pairings that describe animals and what they do (e.g., *fish swim*), between objects and their attributes (e.g., *red rose*), and so forth. In addition, words that occur together in familiar phrases or sequences are likely to be closely associated (e.g., *bread and butter, one, two, three*). If a hearing-impaired child cannot identify a word in a sentence, the child might be able to guess what it is simply by reference to other words that also have been spoken. For example, in the sentence fragment about the *carpenter*, we might reasonably guess that the missing item is *nail*, as this word often is spoken with the word *hammer(ed)*, and in addition, the word *nail* describes an object that carpenters use in their work.

A hearing-impaired child can benefit from learning to use the rules of grammar to interpret unclear messages or to predict another person's spoken responses. A teacher or therapist can direct the child's attention to word order in sentences, and relations between words and phrases. These are sometimes described as *syntactic* and *semantic* communication activities.

Word order

Grammatical rules specify the order in which a person can speak words to communicate. For example, we may say, "The grass is green", "Is the grass green?", or perhaps "____ green the grass is!" We are not likely to say "grass the green is!" if we want to communicate easily with other people who speak our language.

If a hearing-impaired child misperceives one or more words in a sentence, the perceptual gaps can be filled by making informed "guesses" based on what people often say. A particular child, however, may have difficulty making sense of unclear sentence fragments. The child may not realize, for example, that a noun or perhaps a verb was misperceived, and so the child cannot correct the perceptual error by "filling in" an appropriate word type. Remedial activities could include:

- giving the child practice in completing message fragments
- helping the child become more aware of common word order, word forms, and idioms
- demonstrating how to use a linguistic framework to recover incomplete messages.

You could start by presenting the main part of each sentence audio-visually, but with key words spoken as a "bzzz", without voice, or behind a barrier such as your hand, card, or cloth (see figure 4.6). Another activity could involve presenting sentences in printed form, with particular words or phrases shown as blank spaces (Jennings 1995) (see sentence frame examples below). Item difficulty can be varied by creating sentence frames that differ in complexity. The child is asked to "guess" what might have been spoken during the gap. For example, a sentence frame such as "____ is not here!" should elicit a noun or noun phrase. Acceptable responses might be "*Norm* is not here!" or "*the cat* is not here!" In this exercise, the specific words used to fill the gaps are not important.

Some sentence frames used in syntactic practice

___ is not here.

___ is ___.

I am ___, and you are ___.

After ___, we ___.

How many ___?

Does it ___ ?

Where is ___?

___ are not in the ___.

The ___ was ___ by the ___.

Word/phrase associations

The rules of word order are not the only linguistic clues that a hearing-impaired child can use to make sense of an unclear message. Words in sentences also tend to be meaningfully related to one another. For example, there is a close association between the two words *birds fly*, which describe a common event, but there is little relation between the two words *birds study*, which describe an improbable event. People recognize close relationships between words due to: (1) frequent pairing of the words themselves in spoken communication (e.g., "Once upon a time ..." or "Go to sleep") and (2) frequent occurrence of the actual events or situations (e.g., *bouncing ball*, or *blue sky*).

Some children may not realize that they can "guess" the identity of unclear parts of a spoken message by considering the semantic relationship to other words or phrases in the utterance; for example, "The girl combed her long blond *eh*." You can show a child that unclear words in sentences or lists can often be identified on the basis of meaningful associations with other words and phrases in the sequence that were confidently perceived.

It may be beneficial to use activities that demonstrate the close association between types of words (e.g., *short, long, tall, fat*); words in categories (e.g., *farm animals, breakfast foods*); words in common phrases; a noun phrase and verb phrase in the same sentence; or even successive sentences in a narrative (see examples of semantic relationships below). You may ask a child to fill gaps in spoken or printed sequences of words, phrases, or sentences (see A. Lists of words on page 121) (Jeffers & Barley 1971; Chermak 1981; Jennings 1995). This task can often be completed on the basis of relationships between items in categories (e.g., *car, bus, train*, ____), between people and what they frequently say or do (e.g., "Plumbers fix broken ____"), or between adjectives, nouns, and verbs (e.g., "The hungry

____ meowed"). Alternatively, you may choose not to show gaps simply as blank spaces, but as likely perceptual errors; for example, "Jane bought a pair of brown leather *candles* to match her new dress". In this instance, the child must replace the incorrect word with the most likely alternative.

Examples of semantic relationships

A. Groups of associated words (Entwisle 1966)

short: long, tall, fat

sheep: wool, lamb, animal

loud: soft, noise, quiet

dark: light, night, black

chair: table, sit, seat

thirsty: water, drink, dry

hand: foot, arm, finger

smooth: rough, soft, hard

bitter: sweet, sour, taste

needle: thread, pin, sharp

B. Words in familiar categories

farm animals: cow, horse, sheep, chicken

hand tools: hammer, screwdriver, saw, file

household furniture: table, chair, bed, desk

C. Common phrases containing associated words (Alyeshmerni & Taubr 1975)

a cup of coffee   bacon and eggs

rich or poor   eat like a pig

bread and butter   a bowl of cereal

slow as a turtle   sticks and stones

law and order   stubborn as a mule

D. Redundant/predictive sentences (Kalikow et al., 1977)

Football is a dangerous sport.   Stir your coffee with a spoon.

On the beach we play in the sand.   We saw a flock of wild geese.

A bear has a thick coat of fur.   This key won't fit in the lock.

The little girl cuddled her doll.   A rose bush has sharp thorns.

We heard the ticking of the clock.   The dealer shuffled the cards.

E. Successive sentences in a narrative (Streng et al., 1955; Jeffers & Barley 1971; Prince 1982)

The itsy bitsy spider climbed up the water spout.

Down came the rain and washed the spider out.

Out came the sun and dried up all the rain.

And the itsy bitsy spider climbed up the spout again.

The difficulty of these tasks will depend on the specific phrases or sentences, which may differ greatly in their redundancy (Kalikow et al., 1977) (see B. Sentence frames below). For example, in the sentence, "Please find *finial* in the dictionary" the words that surround *finial* tell us only that it is a word, but they give us no clue to its meaning. Moreover, a hearing-impaired child may misperceive not only important "key" words, but also the surrounding phrase or sentence context, which can lead to more complex identification errors. For example, a hearing-impaired young adult misperceived the sentence, "I parked the car at my house" as "I picked up a cat and mouse". She said the error occurred because she identified the words *my house* confidently as *mouse*, the words *I parked* as *I picked*, and simply forced the remainder of the sentence into this self-created framework.

Examples of activities used in semantic practice

A. Lists: child supplies missing word

giraffe, elephant, ____, lion, chimpanzee, zebra

shirt, coat, boots, belt, hat, ____ , scarf, gloves

steak, ____, bacon, fish, hamburger, chicken

apricot, pineapple, ____, watermelon, orange

chair, lamp, bed, bookcase, table, couch, ____

wrench, screwdriver, pliers, ____, saw, drill

B. Sentence frames: child supplies missing word

Highly predictable:

He was so angry, he slammed the ____.

My car has another flat ____.

Please wipe your ____ on the mat.

The little girl clapped her ____.

Dig the ____ over here, by this bush.

He baked a ____ for her birthday.

Would you like another cup of ____?

Moderately predictable:

My dog won't eat ____.

We've just moved to South ____.

She and her husband have ____ children.

He gave the ____ bicycle to the boy.

This computer has a broken ____.

We fed some bread to the ____.

We saw ____ in the barn.

Not very predictable:

We often talked about the ____.

I just bought a ____.

He didn't know about the ____.

Please don't ask me about the ____.

> I've never heard of a ____.
> Do you have a ____?
> We couldn't remember the name of the ____.

Conversational sequences

Conversation consists of an exchange of ideas by two (or more) people. To avoid confusion, the participants agree on generally accepted "rules". These rules include:

- each person should be truthful, informative, topic-relevant, and unambiguous (Grice 1975)
- each person should have a regular opportunity to talk
- only one person should talk at any particular time
- procedures should indicate when it is the other person's turn to talk (Clark & Clark 1977)
- speaking turns begin and end according to social conventions such as eye contact, facial expression, gesture, posture, voice level and pitch, pause, prompting, and so forth (Duncan 1972; Sacks et al., 1974; Weiner & Goodenough 1977).

What one person says often produces predictable responses in the other person. A common example is the result of saying, "Good morning!" Usually the other person will greet you in return. If you ask a specific question, the other person might answer in a predictable way (see examples below). A hearing-impaired child who is aware of contingent sequences like these can anticipate the form of a message that is spoken in response to what the child said first.

Examples of "contingent sequences"

Greeting: "Hello, Max!"
Greeting: "Hi, Jenni!"
Question: "How're you going to school tomorrow?"
Answer: "Oh, I'll probably ride my new bike."
Request: "Could you stop at my house?"
Grant/refusal: "OK. It's on my way!"
Offer: "Should I wait at the corner?"
Acceptance/rejection: "Nah! I'll come at 8:00 and ring the bell."
Compliment: "Your new bike looks great!"
Acceptance/rejection: "Thanks! I got it for my birthday."
Statement: "Slow down! You're going too fast for me!"
Acknowledgement: "Uh ..."
or

> **Agreement/disagreement**: "It's not too fast for me!"
> or
> **Elaboration**: "I'll be in trouble if I'm late for school again!"
> or
> **Question**: "Are you getting tired?"

It may be beneficial for a hearing-impaired child to practice anticipating the form and content of responses to different types of "initiators". For example, you could make a list of conversational topics and a list of related statements or questions (see table 7.1). You then ask the child to speak an item from the list; for example, pets: "Did you remember to feed the fish?" and to predict your possible responses (e.g., "Yes, I did" or "No, I forgot!").

Table 7.1 **Topics and statements used in conversational practice**

Topic/child's statement	Expected response
Weather: "I think it will rain…"	(" ")
Illness: "Everyone in our family has the flu!"	(" ")
Birthday: "My birthday is in April!"	(" ")
Lunch: "I'd like a sandwich."	(" ")
School: "I ride the bus to school."	(" ")
Breakfast: "I'll make the toast!"	(" ")
Television: "I want to watch cartoons!"	(" ")
Babies: "My little brother is two years old."	(" ")

Contingent conversational sequences differ in their associative strength, however, and the ability to predict a response may therefore vary. It can be especially difficult to predict the response to a *statement* (e.g., a description, opinion, or expression of feeling). Possible responses to a statement include an acknowledgement, agreement/disagreement, elaboration, or even a question. For example, if a child wakes up in the morning and moans pathetically, "I feel sick …", this statement may elicit a wide variety of responses. It could evoke a very sympathetic response from his mother: "Oh, you poor baby … you should stay in bed today." The child's mother, however, could also respond to his expression of discomfort by scolding him: "You silly boy! I told you not to eat so much cake at the party last night!" When this kind of statement is made, the child is expressing a personal attitude, feeling, or opinion, and is essentially inviting his mother to respond in a similar way. It has been suggested that making a statement demonstrates trust in the communication partner's interactive style (Luterman 1984). But responses to statements are often hard to predict.

THE A:SQUE PROCEDURE

Most conversational turns contain an "initiator" and a spoken response (Erber & Lind 1994; see figure 4.2). The *type* of initiator strongly influences the number of possible responses and thus the intelligibility of the spoken sentence that follows (see Miller et al., 1951; Sumby & Pollack 1954). Generally speaking, the relatively predictable response that follows a Yes/No question is easier to identify than is the unrestricted response to a statement (see Erber 1996). Table 7.2 gives examples of some common initiators used in the A:SQUE procedure.

Table 7.2 **Examples of questions and statements used in the A:SQUE procedure (Erber 1996)**

Yes/No questions
Are you afraid of spiders?
Are you a vegetarian?
Have you been to a wedding?
Are you a good singer?
Do you like to eat olives?
Choice questions
Would you like soup or salad?
Would you like chocolate or vanilla ice-cream?
Did you fix your bike, or is it still broken?
Is your dance class today or tomorrow?
Would you like chicken or fish for dinner?
Information-eliciting questions
What year were you born?
How many coins do you have?
Which television channel do you usually watch?
How old is the big tree near your house?
Where's the nearest post office?

Table 7.2 **continued**

Opinion-eliciting questions
Why do we have traffic lights?
Why is she your favorite teacher?
How do you feel about camping?
Why are people afraid of worms?
How did they repair the window?
Statements
I like to read cookbooks.
My mother saves old Christmas cards.
I wash my hair every morning.
Some babies cry a lot.
My cat had kittens.

The A:SQUE (Answers to Statements and Questions) procedure is designed to:

1 show a child that the type of spoken initiator (stimulus) can affect the intelligibility of a communication partner's response
2 demonstrate differences between limiting and non-limiting initiators
3 show how the child's conscious choice of initiating sentences can influence the ease of communication.

Turn-initiators, such as questions, requests, and statements, can be used in many different interactive procedures (Erber 1996). The following A:SQUE activities are generally suitable for older children with reasonable reading skills. You can provide interactive practice with or without visible cues, and add background noise or other distractions to increase difficulty.

This therapeutic approach, incorporating self-discovery and analysis rather than instruction, promotes learning and retention of many problem-solving (and problem-avoidance) principles.

Activity 1: Con-sequence

The goals of this activity are:

1 to help the child recognize that there are different types of questions and statements
2 to show that some initiators greatly limit the form and content of a person's response, but that other initiators limit the response only by topic.

The child speaks initiators from the A:SQUE lists; for example, five Yes/No questions, five choice questions, five Wh- questions, and so forth. You reply appropriately to each initiator (e.g., child: "When does the store open?" and you reply: "at 9:30"). The child repeats each response, and you verify correct identification. If difficulty occurs, both apply clarification strategies until the child can identify your response. After this practice, you and the child discuss how each type of initiator can affect the intelligibility of your response.

Activity 2: Con-tingent

The goals of this activity are to:
1 simulate the various stimulus-response sequences that occur in real conversations
2 help the child become aware of differences and similarities between particular initiator types.

Initiators of various types (e.g., 20 yes/no, 20 choice, etc.) are printed on small cards, one to a card. A similar number of blank cards (e.g., 20) are also included. The deck is shuffled and placed face down on the table. The child takes the top card, speaks the question/statement, and you respond appropriately. When a blank card appears, this signals *you* to take the next card and speak the question/statement to the child. This reversal of roles simulates the child's loss of control of the topic during conversation. If communication difficulty occurs, both you and the child apply clarification strategies until the child can identify what you said. Later, you and the child discuss why each spoken answer or initiator was difficult or easy to understand.

Activity 3: Con-sider

The goals of this activity are:
1 to demonstrate that initiators of different types elicit spoken responses that may differ in intelligibility
2 to demonstrate that difficulties can usually be anticipated.

The general procedure for this activity is similar to Activity 2 (Con-tingent), already described, but now the child is required to predict the difficulty of identifying your response *before* you speak. That is, the child first considers the potential difficulty of understanding your response to each initiator, and sorts the cards accordingly into a "Difficult" or "Easy" pile. Then the child speaks the initiators in each pile, listens to your responses, and decides whether the predictions of difficulty were correct. A likely discovery is that your responses to *statements* are often difficult to anticipate and thus difficult to identify.

Activity 4: Con-descending

The goals are to:

1 help the child discover a hierarchy of initiators that may influence the intelligibility of a person's spoken response

2 help the child learn to use lower-level initiators adaptively.

A list of *statements* on various topics is prepared. When the child speaks a statement from this list, you reply appropriately. The child must then create and ask a descending series of *questions* related to the topic: opinion, information, choice, yes/no. For example, for the topic *television*:

"I don't watch television very much." (statement from list)

"Why don't you watch television?" (*opinion* question)

"Which programs do you watch?" (*information* question)

"Do you watch the news on Channel 2 or 7?" (*choice* question)

"Did you watch a DVD last night?" (*yes/no* question)

Reply to each initiator appropriately. If communication difficulty occurs, clarification strategies should be applied as necessary, until the child can identify your response. After each group of items, you and the child should discuss the difficulty of communicating at each initiator level.

Activity 5: Con-openers

The goal of this activity is to give the child practice in generating conversation initiators of various types without prompting from printed lists or stimulus cards.

The child is required to "open conversations" in various ways that you request (e.g., "Ask me a choice (this or that) question about *grapefruit!*"; "Now tell me something about *shoes!*"). Reply to each conversation opener appropriately. Provide clarification as necessary until the child can identify your response. Note the amount of time the child takes to create and present each type of initiator and discuss this with the child.

CONVERSATION REPAIR

In many auditory communication programs, a hearing-impaired child acquires listening skills through a close relationship with an attentive and accommodating adult (e.g., a parent or therapist), who insures that conversational interaction is maintained. Not all conversation partners, however, can or will provide the same degree of cooperation. When a misunderstanding occurs, a conversation can become confusing and break down. In order to communicate with a wide range of conversation partners, a hearing-impaired child will need to learn to play the role of "conversation manager".

Sources of difficulty

There are many reasons why a conversation may become confusing and disordered (see table 7.3). The source of the difficulty could be one of the communicators, the topic, or the situation. It is important for the child to be able to correctly identify the cause of each breakdown when it happens; for example, the listening system, unclear speech, message complexity, ambiguity, or even a combination of causes. This means that the hearing-impaired child must be able to analyze the conversation, the situation, and the environment for potential sources of confusion.

Table 7.3 **Potential sources of confusion in conversation**

Child's hearing and linguistic skills	Cannot detect, discriminate, or identify units of speech
	Does not recognize own hearing limitations
	Malfunction of hearing aids/cochlear implants
	Poor meta-communication ability
	Inattention
	Fatigue or illness
Communication partner's speech	Rapid syllable rate
	Voice level too low, fluctuating, decreasing
	Voice pitch too high, fluctuating, increasing
	Unclear articulation
	Foreign or regional accent (e.g., unusual prosody/intonation/stress)
	Mouth/face obscured by hand, hair, or object
Communication partner's message	Unfamiliar topic or sudden topic shift
	Uncommon words, technical terms, jargon
	Colloquial expressions
	Long sentences
	Complex syntax (e.g., passive verb, embedded clause)
	Too many sentences presented in succession (e.g., long narrative)
	Unfamiliar with clarification methods
	Lack of cooperation
Conversational environment	Long distance between the communicators
	High noise level
	High reverberation (echo)
	Low illumination level
	Glare from reflecting objects
	Visual distractions

Conversation difficulty or breakdown can arise from errors in anticipation or perception. Often the child will realize that a misunderstanding has occurred, but not know why. The child may appear confused or request help in a vague, non-specific way (see A. Non-specific request examples below). Repetition alone by the communication partner may not be a sufficient remedy. It is generally more effective for the child to identify the cause of the confusion, and request a specific, appropriate type of clarification (Caissie & Wilson 1995; Lloyd 1999) (see B. Specific request examples below).

Examples of A. non-specific and B. specific requests for clarification in response to conversational difficulty

A. Non-specific requests

Difficulty	*Clarification request*
Reduced volume:	"What?"
Increased rate:	"I missed some of that."
Long/complex:	"Excuse me … what was that?"
Turned away:	"I didn't hear you."
Combinations of above:	"What did you say?"

B. Specific requests

Difficulty	*Clarification request*
Reduced volume:	"Please talk louder."
Increased rate:	"Please slow down a little."
Long/complex:	"I didn't hear the last part … "
Turned away:	"Please look at me when you speak."
Combinations of above:	"Did you say you live in … Coburg?"

Problem-solving

A general *problem-solving* approach can be used to repair most common conversational difficulties (Erber 1996). There are several steps in the process (Demorest 1986). This approach to conversational problem-solving may be difficult for a younger child (Cohen 2006), but within the capability of an older child.

Steps in conversational problem-solving

1 recognize that conversational difficulty has occurred
2 identify the source of the difficulty
3 request or apply a strategy to overcome the problem
4 judge the effectiveness of the strategy
5 confirm that the message was received correctly (e.g., "Did you say …?")
6 if the message was received correctly, continue the conversation
7 if the strategy did not resolve the difficulty, consider why it failed (e.g., misjudged source of difficulty; strategy not applied correctly)

8 request/apply the original strategy correctly, or
9 request/apply an alternative strategy
10 return to step 4.

ACTIVITIES TO PROMOTE REQUESTS FOR CLARIFICATION

A hearing-impaired child may benefit from preparation for conversation difficulty. A variety of specific practice activities can be used to help the child learn how to reliably identify common sources of conversational confusion, describe them to a communication partner, and request clarification. Although natural interaction with a parent, relative, or friend is real and motivating, it may not provide sufficient concentrated practice to enable the child to communicate confidently with an unfamiliar or less cooperative partner. When interacting naturally with a highly familiar communication partner, the relationship, topic, and situation often provide sufficient meaningful context to enable the child to understand a perceptually unclear message *without* requesting clarification. It may also be easier to bluff, delay, and/or wait for further information or spontaneous clarification provided by the familiar partner.

There are many ways to encourage problem-solving and provide specific practice to a hearing-impaired child (Lloyd 1999). The following activities are just two examples.

Elicitation of clarification requests

This activity uses QUEST?AR materials (Erber 1996, (see pp. 88–90) to give a child practice in recognizing sources of difficulty. The adult responds to the child's questions with various sources of perceptual difficulty that are intentionally superimposed on the spoken responses (see table 7.4). The child must identify the type of difficulty and request appropriate clarification from the adult until each response is understood.

Table 7.4 **Some ways to make communication difficult**

Speech	speak with high voice pitch
	speak rapidly
	speak softly
	reduce voice level at the end of a sentence

Table 7.4 **continued**

	reduce acoustic clarity of articulation
	reduce visible clarity of articulation
	obscure the mouth
	move, tilt, or turn the head while speaking
	use distracting gestures
Language	rare words, colloquialisms, or jargon
	inverted sentences
	long, complicated sentences
	inanimate subjects
	embedded clauses
	passive verb forms

Before you begin, write the specific speech/language difficulty that you intend to apply in response to each QUEST?AR question (e.g., soft voice, rapid speech, complex sentence). Then superimpose these difficulties on your speech or language as you answer the child's questions.

The child's tasks are:

1   to identify each answer
2   to identify the difficulty that you imposed on that answer
3   to request appropriate clarification
4   to identify the modified answer.

Note the degree of success in identifying and responding to each imposed difficulty (see table 7.5), and discuss the results with the child. In the example shown below, the results indicate that the child was unable to recognize sentence complexity as a source of confusion.

Table 7.5 **Identification of sources of auditory difficulty during a QUEST?AR practice session**

Source of difficulty				
	Soft voice	**Rapid speech**	**Unclear speech**	**Complex sentence**
Difficulty identified?				
Yes	4	4	3	0
No	1	1	2	5

Referential communication

A typical referential communication task involves presenting an ambiguous situation or complex message without visible cues. The child must follow the instructions or respond appropriately. The child is allowed and encouraged to request additional spoken information or clarification whenever misunderstanding occurs (Ibertsson et al., 2009). Barrier games (Chapter 5) and telephone communication (Chapter 6) can both be used to implement the referential communication method.

In one example of a referential communication task (Lloyd 1999), various small objects are placed in front of the child (e.g., *red/yellow/blue spoons, big/small cups*). The adult selects a picture illustrating a combination of objects, but does not show it to the child. The adult requests the child reproduce what is shown in the picture without giving an important detail, for example, "Put the blue spoon in the cup" (omitting the *size* of the cup). The child must request additional information in order to complete the task, for example "in the *big* cup?" Later, the adult shows the picture to the child to verify that the spoken message was identified correctly.

In another example (Lloyd 1991, 1992), identical maps are placed before the adult and child including the location of several landmarks such as houses, garages, trees, bridges, etc. A desired route for travel is shown on the adult's map. The adult speaks route instructions but omits important details ("First, go to the *garage*."). The child must trace the route, and request clarification when the message or its meaning cannot be understood ("Did you say garage? Which one ... the *brown* garage?"). When the activity is completed, the two maps are compared to verify that the correct route was identified.

SUMMARY

This chapter has described various ways that situational, interpersonal, and sequential contexts can help a child to accurately receive spoken messages. Language-use strategies based on syntactic and semantic contexts were suggested to help a child identify unclear sentences. Conversation repair strategies, including problem-solving methods and clarification-request activities, were also described in detail.

CHAPTER 8

Speech development

For an infant with normal hearing, learning to hear, decode and produce the patterns of spoken language are natural processes that begin at birth. The infant listens to the speech of others, imitates what is heard, and uses these sounds to communicate. When a young hearing-impaired child receives hearing aids or cochlear implants, this is an opportunity to acquire spoken language through listening.

DEVELOPMENTAL STAGES

Most children with normal hearing pass through a sequence of developmental stages as they learn to generate acoustic features, sound sequences, and meaningful utterances of spoken language (Oller 1980; Locke 1993). These stages include:

- reflex sounds/vocal signals, such as cooing and crying, that express pleasure or discomfort
- urgent calls that are intended to influence others – e.g., requests for attention, demands and protests
- babbling/vocal play – i.e., production of syllabic patterns that include vowel-like sounds combined with consonant-like sounds
- approximations to the speech patterns of adults
- first words – i.e., meaningful linkage of speech-sound patterns with people, objects, situations, or experiences
- simple two-word combinations – e.g., noun + verb
- simple sentences
- interactive conversational sequences.

Although some vocalizations such as crying and babbling appear to be innate processes, children with normal hearing develop most of the above skills mainly from *listening*. They listen both to the speech of others and to the sounds they produce themselves. At first, they generate a wide variety of speech-like sounds, but soon learn to limit their production to sounds that they hear others use. They also listen to their own vocalizations through an "auditory feedback loop", through which they judge the accuracy of their utterances and adjust them accordingly.

The auditory system is an ideal mechanism for perception and processing of spoken language (Stackhouse & Wells 1997; Pickett 1999). Experience has shown that many children with impaired hearing can develop clear speech and fluent spoken language when an auditory approach is used, especially if the following conditions are met (Tobey et al., 1994; Yoshinaga-Itano 1998; Pollack et al., 1997; Flexer 1999; Geers et al., 2011):

- the child's hearing loss is detected early
- an appropriate personal listening system is fitted early and maintained in good working condition
- auditory communication and learning is introduced early
- clear and consistent spoken language is provided in contexts that are familiar and meaningful to the child
- listening experiences occur at a near distance in a good acoustic environment
- the child receives social, emotional, and communicative support from family members, teachers, and therapists.

A hearing-impaired child who receives hearing aids or cochlear implants early in life and regularly listens to his/her own speech, and the speech of others, can develop spoken language through a process similar to that of a child with normal hearing (Ertmer et al., 2007; Tait et al., 2007). In some cases, the stages of speech acquisition may be delayed, however, and progress may be slower. The child may continue to produce deviant speech patterns or omit/misarticulate particular speech sounds.

RELATION BETWEEN SPEECH PERCEPTION AND PRODUCTION

The intelligibility of a child's speech is related in a general way to the child's ability to perceive his/her own speech and the speech of others (Boothroyd 1984; Miyamoto et al., 1996; Calmels et al., 2004). Figure 8.1 shows the open-set auditory sentence-identification scores of a group of hearing-impaired children as a function of the number of years they have used cochlear implants. The diagram also shows their speech intelligibility ratings over the same period of time. For these children, auditory speech perception and speech intelligibility are seen to increase similarly as listening experience accumulates. Results like this also have been obtained from children who have used hearing aids for many years (Boothroyd 1984; Eisenberg 2007).

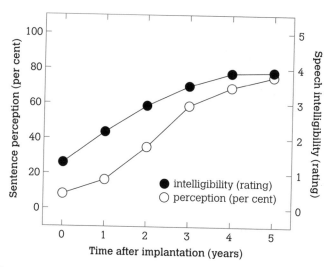

Figure 8.1 **Perception and production of speech by 63 hearing-impaired children after cochlear implantation. Data points are group medians (Calmels et al., 2004)**

While some hearing-impaired children learn to produce speech sounds that they cannot hear clearly (Smith 1975; Ling 1989), this is generally the exception rather than the rule. Most hearing-impaired children have persistent difficulty producing speech sounds and sound patterns that they cannot hear. Large individual differences in speech development have been observed. The reasons include differences:

- in the age at which the child first receives hearing aids or cochlear implants
- in the ability to hear particular speech sounds clearly, even with an optimal personal listening system (neither hearing aids nor cochlear implants restore normal hearing)
- in processing/amplification of hearing aids or cochlear implants that may affect the prominence of particular speech features (Boothroyd et al., 1988; Tomblin et al., 2008)
- in the amount and type of spoken input, therapy, or instruction that the child receives
- in the speech and language clarity of regular communication partners
- in the distance at which auditory communication regularly occurs
- in incidental learning from nearby communicators due to differences in "effective hearing distance"
- in the amount of background noise and echo in home and school environments
- between children in their attention to visible cues and reliance on these cues for learning speech and language

- between children in the amount of speech perception and production experience received before acquisition of hearing aids or cochlear implants (O'Donoghue et al., 1999).

A hearing-impaired child's progress as an auditory communicator is usually closely monitored and assessed. It is important to remember that the results of such assessments can be influenced by the experience of the listener (McGarr 1983; Most & Shurgi 1993). Speech may be assessed by:

- rating its overall intelligibility (Shriberg & Kwiatkowski 1982; Levitt et al., 1987)
- measuring the percentage of key words or syllables that can be identified by a listener (Blamey et al., 2001; Flipsen & Colvard 2006)
- specifying speech sounds that are produced correctly or incorrectly (Ling 1976; Tobey et al., 2003)
- analyzing its acoustic characteristics in detail (Monsen 1978, 1983b; Uchanski & Geers 2003).

COMMON SPEECH ERRORS

Even if a child has received appropriate listening devices and engaged in auditory communication from an early age, the child may still produce spoken language that is not completely intelligible to all people all of the time. Children generally exhibit expressive errors that are a function of their auditory abilities, personal listening systems, and years of listening experience (Boothroyd 1984; Abraham 1989; Tye-Murray et al., 1995a, 1995b; Calmels et al., 2004; Most & Peled 2007).

What follows is a brief overview of the speech behavior of hearing-impaired children, based on available observations, research, and clinical test results.

Temporal (timing) patterns

Speech deviations may occur in the rhythm, stress pattern, syllable rate, or overall duration of a sentence (Hudgins & Numbers 1942; Markides 1983; Maassen & Povel 1985; Ling 1989). Many of these difficulties are related to inappropriate regulation of the breath stream (Nickerson 1975; Whitehead 1983). Timing variations that can affect the intelligibility of an utterance include:

- producing syllables too slowly
- not differentiating between stressed (strong) and unstressed (weak) syllables
- improperly inserting or filling pauses in connected speech (e.g., speaking a syllable without voice)
- grouping syllables inappropriately.

Voice pitch and quality

A child produces voice when exhaled air passes through the vocal folds and causes them to vibrate. Voice pitch is related to the rate of airflow and the mass/elasticity of the vocal folds. There are two main types of voice pitch deviation:

1 inappropriate average pitch – e.g., pitch typically too high
2 inappropriate pitch *change* – e.g., monotone voice, sudden pitch variations, inappropriate intonation contour.

The voice quality of some hearing-impaired children has also been described as "weak", "breathy", "harsh", or "tense", all of which are generally attributed to inappropriate positioning of the vocal folds during speech (Calvert, 1962; Ling, 1989).

Articulation

Articulation errors may be present in the speech of hearing-impaired children. Typical consonant-articulation errors include:

- failure to distinguish unvoiced/voiced consonants that are produced at the same place in the mouth, especially the stop-plosives (e.g., /t, d/)
- mis-articulation of speech sounds that contain high-frequency energy (e.g., /s, ʃ/)
- distortion/omission of consonants (particularly in final position in a word)
- difficulty in producing appropriate transitions within a sequence of speech sounds (Levitt 1971; Ling 1989).

The speech of some hearing-impaired children is characterized by inappropriate nasality, resulting from poor control of the soft palate (velum). Excessive nasality can cause the voiced stops /b, d, g/ to sound like their nasal counterparts /m, n, ŋ/. Some children also have difficulty producing consonant clusters that contain nasal consonants, such as /nt, nd, mp/ (Ling 1976).

Some hearing-impaired children do not position their tongues precisely enough to produce appropriate vowel qualities (Ling 1989). A child may produce a vowel that is imprecise, nasalized, or fluctuates in quality. Researchers have reported a reduced frequency range of both the first and second formants in the vowels of some hearing-impaired children (Monsen & Shaughnessy 1978; Ozbic & Kogovšek 2010). This can make it difficult for a listener to clearly distinguish different vowel sounds that a child produces. A limited range of vowel articulation may also impair the intelligibility of adjacent consonants whose correct identification depends on appropriate vowel-formant transitions (Monsen 1978).

"Linguistic" errors

Omission of unstressed syllables or verb endings is common in the spoken language of some hearing-impaired children. Although these errors are usually described as deficiencies in expressive "language", they probably result from a child's *auditory* limitations. Verb endings such as -s, -ing, and many other weak syllables can be difficult for a hearing-impaired child to hear or see when spoken quickly, and therefore tend to be omitted or used incorrectly in the child's speech. Other brief and acoustically weak language components include articles such as *a* and *the*, unstressed prefixes and suffixes, plural markers, pronouns, and prepositions.

AUDITORY-BASED SPEECH COMMUNICATION ACTIVITIES

Parents, family members, teachers, and therapists can provide enjoyable listening and talking experiences throughout the day, to promote and stimulate the child's development of spoken language (Estabrooks & Birkenshaw-Fleming 2003; Caleffe-Schenck & Baker 2008). Activities could include:

- modeling of spoken language during all daily activities
- rhymes and songs that emphasize particular speech sounds
- reading/listening/speaking games
- modeling of intensity/pitch patterns and the content of words, phrases, and sentences
- emphasis ("highlighting") to elicit appropriate responses
- expansion of the child's utterances to include omitted details
- reinforcement and encouragement of the child's attempts to vocalize and speak.

Adult models of spoken language

Most of a young child's early vocalizations and attempts to communicate are related to:

- the child's needs, wants, and interests
- the child's desire to clarify meaning
- the child's development of relationships.

An adult can easily model spoken language during all daily activities, whenever a young child expresses communicative intent. The child may use a recognizable gesture, posture, or vocalization to express the intended meaning. By modeling an appropriate spoken utterance in each instance, the adult demonstrates the link between spoken language and communication in that context. For example:

- points/vocalizes – "I want ..."
- pushes away/cries/screams – "I don't want ..."

- pulls on highchair/cries – "I'm thirsty/hungry!"
- points/cries/bangs container – "More!"
- shrugs/palms up – "Where's my dolly/teddy/etc.?"
- brings/presents object – "This is my …"
- raises arms/looks up – "Pick me up!"
- brings toy/tugs on leg – "Play with me!"
- attempts to climb on knee – "I want a horsey ride!"
- pushes/crawls/walks away/cries – "Leave me alone!"
- acts manic/is lethargic – "I'm tired."
- complains/rubs eyes/cries – "It's time for sleep!"
- points to bathtub – "It's time for a bath!"
- reaches out to parent – "I want mummy/daddy!"
- giggles, sings, babbles, sits quietly – "I'm happy!"
- cries/is lethargic/doesn't eat – "I'm sick."

Songs and rhymes

Songs and rhymes provide the child with enjoyable experiences while singing/speaking sound patterns (Estabrooks & Birkenshaw-Fleming 2003). Songs and rhymes are fun and maintain the child's interest. They can be introduced in a developmental sequence, with initial emphasis on speech sounds that are typically easier for infants to produce (e.g., /p/), followed by speech sounds that are harder to learn (e.g., /f/) (Caleffe-Schenck & Baker 2008).

Some popular children's songs and rhymes

This little piggy went to market
Baa baa black sheep
Hokey Pokey
Hickory dickory dock
Humpty Dumpty
Little Miss Muffet
Old MacDonald had a farm
Three blind mice

Therapeutic play

An adult can organize sound play, sound games, and other activities with dolls or toys (e.g., *monkey, mouse, monster*), household objects (e.g., *comb, cup, computer*), common words (e.g., *best, nest, rest*), or silly phrases (e.g., *find the furry fox*) that contain specific speech sounds or sound patterns (Caleffe-Schenck & Baker 2008).

These activities provide a young child with opportunities to listen to adult models of spoken language and to practice producing similar utterances.

> **Common play activities that contain the speech sound /b/ (Caleffe-Schenck & Baker 2008)**
>
> Bake a cake.
> String beads.
> Ride your bike.
> Bounce the ball.
> Build with blocks.
> Blow bubbles in the bath.
> Put your toy box in the bedroom.
> Find birds and butterflies in the backyard.

Structured activities

Play activities can be organized that require the child to ask for a toy, describe objects/events, or answer questions (Moog & Geers 1985). Each request, description, or answer can lead to a brief conversation. For example, while reading or acting out a story, an adult could ask the child to describe a picture – "What is the caterpillar doing now?" or could ask a question such as "What happened to the frog?" These activities require spoken responses from the child. The adult and child could also participate in a referential communication task where the child plays the role of speaker and the adult attempts to follow the child's spoken instructions (Lloyd et al., 2005; see Chapter 7 for more details). For an older child, a more natural conversation-based approach may be preferred, where the adult and child discuss topics that reflect the child's current interests.

ADAPTIVE METHODS

Persistent speech errors may require an adaptive approach. The main steps include:

1 engaging the child in play or structured interactive activities that elicit target vocalizations or spoken language from the child (Caleffe-Schenck & Baker 2008)
2 analyzing the child's utterances for errors (e.g., voice, prosody, intonation, articulation, and linguistic details such as plural or verb tense markers)
3 acoustically modeling correct speech
4 asking the child to listen and imitate
5 asking the child to judge the accuracy of imitation
6 judging the accuracy of the child's imitation yourself

7 applying adaptive strategies (acoustic repetition, emphasis, prompting)

8 rewarding the child's successive approximations to correct speech production

9 providing visible cues only if the child experiences persistent difficulty

10 using "fading" techniques to reduce the child's reliance on cues and prompts.

The following adaptive strategies are commonly used (Erber & Greer 1973; Erber 1980b; Caleffe-Schenck & Baker 2008):

- repetition
- clarification
- distortion/exaggeration
- spoken instructions and prompts
- gestural and behavioral prompts
- visual and tactile cues.

A phonological framework for therapy is recommended. This means that the focus of therapy is the child's ability to produce speech-sound contrasts that convey differences in *meaning*, not the child's ability to produce speech sounds in isolation or in unrelated syllables (Abraham 1989). Some examples of phonological processes include adding the sound /s/ after an unvoiced consonant to indicate the plurality of a noun such as *cat*, or producing the sound /t/ after an unvoiced consonant to indicate the past tense of a verb such as *lick*.

Repetition

A child's awareness of acoustic details in speech will vary as a function of the child's attention to the task, intermittent background noise, or other environmental distractions. If conditions are satisfactory, simply repeating the model utterance, followed by the child's imitation, may be sufficient to yield accurate production. If the child was distracted, it can be beneficial to optimize listening conditions before repeating the target item, for example, reduce distance, eliminate background noise, etc.

Clarification

Clarification involves giving increased acoustic prominence to a particular feature as you model the target utterance. For example, the child may have spoken the two syllables of the word *father* with similar stress. You could correct this error by emphasizing the differences in syllable intensity or duration ("FA ther"). If the child omits a pause between clauses, you could correct this timing error by modeling a more prominent silence in the appropriate place to increase the salience of this feature ("When we walked into the room, … everyone turned around"). Or if a child has produced a sentence with a monotonous voice pitch, you could emphasize the changes in intonation as you model the sentence (see list below for more examples).

Some ways to increase acoustic prominence

- raise/lower your voice level
- raise/lower your voice pitch
- increase/reduce your speech rate
- pause before/after a key syllable or word
- articulate more precisely
- increase the duration of a vowel/continuant consonant
- emphasize the contrast within a diphthong
- modify sound quality

You might also use clarification to correct a child's articulatory errors. For example, if the child has produced /fid/ for the word *feet*, you could model the word by increasing the intensity and duration of the noisy burst in the final consonant (/t/). In the case of vowel imprecision or substitution, you could prolong the vowel while your tongue and lips are in the target position. You could also emphasize parts of diphthongs in a similar manner.

If a child has substituted a word (*the zoo > a zoo*) or omitted a word ending (*farmer > farm*), you could provide clarification by producing the item with greater intensity and/or isolating it between brief pauses. For example, the phrase *in ... bus* (incorrect) can be modeled for the child as *in ... **the** ... bus* to demonstrate the correct phrase. It is recommended that you provide all of these acoustic models without visible cues (figure 8.2).

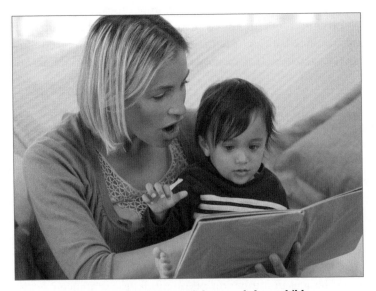

Figure 8.2 **A mother models speech for a child**

This general technique is called "acoustic highlighting" by many educators. It can be very effective in the short term, but if used over a longer period it can create dependency on an adult for speech monitoring and control. To enable the child to incorporate what is learned into his/her own phonological system, the adult should help the child develop a cognitive awareness of what is being highlighted and why. To achieve this goal, the *adult* needs to determine why the omission or error occurred, rather than just model or prompt for self-correction whenever it occurs.

Distortion and exaggeration

Distortion and exaggeration techniques are mainly used to elicit omitted speech sounds that the child is apparently unable to detect or hear clearly. The aim of these techniques is not to model correct acoustic qualities or patterns, but to slightly distort or exaggerate particular speech sounds so that the child can detect them more easily. For example, deliberately producing the sound with a different acoustic quality (e.g., "shoap") is *distortion*. In contrast, simply lengthening a speech sound to make it more prominent (e.g., "sssoap") is an example of *exaggeration*.

You may be able to correct a child's omission of a voiceless stop/plosive or fricative (e.g., /p, t, f, s/) by holding a microphone very close to your mouth (and then close to the child's mouth) to create low-frequency turbulence from the breath stream (Schulte 1978). The child can usually detect the noisy sound that results. Later, although the child receives much less auditory feedback when producing the sound correctly, the child may recall the acoustic image of your distorted utterance.

You may also be able to correct omission of an /s/ by cueing the child with a sound that is more like /ʃ/ in quality, and consequently is more audible to the child. Frequency-transposing hearing aids enhance a child's auditory perception of high-frequency speech sounds by presenting audible (but distorted) lower-frequency surrogates in a similar way (Glista et al., 2009; Kuk et al., 2010)

The principal aim of *distortion* is to make inaudible speech sounds available for phonological representation in the child's internal language, for reference when the child speaks or when the child is engaged in another sound-related task such as reading or spelling. Distortion and exaggeration can help demonstrate to the child that the sounds of speech convey important information. When the child understands this concept, then you can model the correct production acoustically and ask the child to imitate your utterance as he/she listens to its minimal cues.

Spoken instructions and prompts

Some teachers and therapists employ a hierarchy of spoken instructions and prompts to help children modify their speech when an error occurs (Calvert & Silverman 1975). This is sometimes called a "metalinguistic" approach to instruction. Some examples of spoken prompts are:

- "I'm listening carefully, but I still don't understand your speech." (general)
- "You forgot a sound in the last word." (more specific)
- "You forgot to say the /l/ sound in the word *please*." (very specific)

These spoken suggestions not only recommend specific changes, but also remind the child that important information in speech is conveyed by the way that it *sounds* to others.

Gestures and behavioral prompts

Gestures also can be used to direct the child's attention to acoustic patterns in speech, such as pitch change, pause, and stress, or to point out less prominent speech features such as voicing, nasality, stop/plosive, or frication. Gestural prompts can even be organized into a "phonetic cue" system to indicate voicing, nasality, or tongue position (Schulte 1978). It is much more common, however, to use natural and spontaneous hand movements to convey rhythm and emphasis in speech.

Gestural prompts are also commonly used in conjunction with acoustic modeling. For example, you could model two different versions of a word for comparison, that is, your correct production and the child's incorrect production. A natural gestural prompt would be to point to the person who spoke as you reproduce each version, "I said *ribbon* … you said *rimmbon*".

You can easily indicate pitch change by raising or lowering your hand. You can indicate an intensity error by cupping your hand behind your ear (i.e., "too soft") or by covering your ear with your hand (i.e., "too loud"). Natural gestures also are commonly used for "please repeat", "stop", "listen", and so forth. These familiar gestures refer to the *acoustic* nature of speech, although they produce no sound themselves.

Another behavioral approach, described by Lloyd (1999), is to use referential communication activities (see Chapter 7) to demonstrate to a child that his/her expressive errors can lead to significant errors in another person's response behavior. This prompts the child to clarify or self-correct in order to achieve a positive result.

Visual and tactile cues

A child may continue to produce speech errors in spite of acoustic modeling and a variety of adaptive strategies. If you conclude that this is the result of the child's auditory limitations, you may decide to provide additional sensory information in the form of visual or tactile cues.

If a purely auditory approach has not been successful, the therapist can demonstrate correct speech with the mouth uncovered, while the child looks and listens. Speech should be presented without over-articulation of visible mouth movements. Providing visual cues can be effective for a child who persists in substituting one speech sound for another, for example, the child produces /kIp/ for the spoken word *tip*. First, model the word with acoustic cues only. Then, speak the word with the mouth uncovered, providing a visual prompt for the initial place of tongue articulation. Then, cover your mouth and repeat the word before asking the child to imitate. This therapeutic method, where the target item is first spoken with the mouth covered, then with a visual prompt, and then again with the mouth covered, has been called an "auditory sandwich" (A > AV > A) by some educators. The aim is to link the child's articulatory behavior to what the child can hear.

Children with poor auditory skills may benefit from feeling the output of a hand-held tactile vibrator, to compare the vibro-tactile pattern of your model utterance with their own pattern of imitation (see Appendix 2). This tactile technique is most effective for correcting deviant speech *prosody*, such as inappropriate speech rate or syllable stress (Erber 1978, 1982; Schulte 1978), but more subtle distinctions can also be demonstrated. Some children can learn to distinguish a harsh, "rough", or loud voice from a normal, "smooth", or soft voice. It also is possible to indicate the omission or substitution of a speech sound with this technique, for example, *pencil* versus *pen*, or *button* versus *but*. Feel the speech contrasts first, to establish which distinctions in speech are likely to be available to the child through the vibro-tactile device, and which are not. Then model the correct pattern with your mouth obscured, before the child attempts to produce the utterance. The child feels both speech patterns through the tactile vibrator and judges their similarities and differences.

Practical tips

While interacting with the child, ensure that the child listens at a near distance in a good acoustic environment. With regular listening practice and experience, most children can learn to self-monitor and self-correct through an auditory feedback process. Typically, a child learns to quickly hear the more prominent differences between his/her own speech and an adult's model. More practice is usually needed, however, to develop awareness of more subtle acoustic differences.

During a therapy session, an adult will usually feel comfortable correcting the child's speech. If the child has spoken *spontaneously*, however, to share a feeling, express a point of view, or to give/get information, the child's desire is for immediate communication. On these occasions, if the child's intended meaning is apparent, the adult may choose *not* to apply speech/language correction, or to do so cautiously, so as not to disrupt the conversational exchange.

Auditory communication over the telephone (without visible cues) is useful for demonstrating to a child why acoustically intelligible speech is important. A child who recognizes the benefits of auditory communication will allow an adult to briefly interrupt a casual conversation to model parts that are considered incorrect or deviant, and will try repeatedly to match the sound quality of a model utterance.

A careful therapist will continually assess the situation, however, to determine when to emphasize auditory speech instruction and when to simply converse in a natural manner. These decisions will depend on each child's personality, listening skills, and learning style.

Fading

When you use any of the strategies or prompts described in this chapter, be sure to complete the activity by gradually withdrawing the supplementary information and returning to a normal acoustic model. This training technique has been called "fading" by psychologists. Your aim should be to transfer the child's speech monitoring and phonologic processing to the auditory domain, rather than to increase the child's dependence on the compensatory strategies or non-acoustic (visual, tactile) prompts that you have provided. Ultimately, the aim is to help the hearing-impaired child become competent and confident in using hearing aids/cochlear implants and his/her auditory system for expression and self-monitoring of spoken language.

SUMMARY

An auditory approach to speech development is most effective if applied early and consistently, after a child receives hearing aids or cochlear implants. An adult can use acoustic modeling to help a child recognize and correct expressive errors through listening and self-monitoring. A variety of therapeutic strategies are available: repetition, exaggeration, distortion, spoken instruction, and gestural prompting. Supplementary information can be provided, if necessary, in the form of visual or tactile cues. The benefit obtained from each method will depend on the child's listening skills.

CHAPTER 9

Communication partners

Communication partners such as parents, teachers, and friends play a primary role in the speech and language development of a hearing-impaired child. Regular interaction with others is vital to the child's development of spoken language and social competence (Simmons-Martin & Rossi 1990; Simser 1999; Cole & Flexer 2011). The child is likely to acquire auditory skills most easily when communication partners produce spoken language that is consistently audible, visible, and clear.

Many factors contribute to the clarity of a communication partner's speech. Examples include voice pitch, loudness, syllable rate, lip/tongue positions, and facial movements. Speakers can differ greatly in all of these characteristics (Picheny et al., 1985, 1986; Uchanski 2005).

Adult speakers usually listen to themselves as they talk, and use this acoustic feedback to judge their own intelligibility. They may repeat words or phrases, raise their voice level, or exaggerate if they feel their spoken message was not intelligible (Lane & Tranel 1971). People usually do not watch themselves as they talk, however, and therefore lack experience in judging their mouth and tongue visibility.

Various non-speech factors also contribute to the intelligibility of a spoken message. In general, easily understood messages are brief, contain familiar vocabulary and simple language, and fit the situation and conversational context. That is, *what* a person says and *how* or *when* the person says it can affect intelligibility.

Nearly all adults with normal hearing can speak clearly enough to converse with other adults who have normal hearing. Some adults, however, do not speak clearly enough to communicate easily with a child or adult with a significant hearing impairment (Kricos & Lesner 1982; Picheny et al., 1985, 1986; Gagné et al., 1994).

The input that a child receives through impaired hearing, hearing aids/cochlear implants, and/or lipreading may be very different from what the adult spoke. In addition, the child may have neither the linguistic skills nor the life experiences to reconstruct the spoken message and appreciate the idea expressed. Thus speech intelligibility depends not only on the message and how it is spoken, but also on who is listening and looking (Carney 1986).

As the result of trial-and-error, some adults (e.g., the parents of a hearing-impaired child) develop clear speech and language. Their progress may be slow, however, for the following reasons:

- adults cannot hear their own speech as a hearing-impaired child hears it, and thus cannot judge how it sounds to the child
- adults cannot see themselves while talking, and thus cannot judge how they look to the child
- children may not provide enough specific feedback regarding audibility, visibility, or language clarity to help adults modify their communication behavior and improve intelligibility.

TRADITIONAL COMMUNICATION PARTNER TRAINING

Productive communication with a hearing-impaired child requires knowledge, skill, clarity, and patience. Parents and other communication partners can improve their communication skills through structured training (Picheny et al., 1985; Payton et al., 1994; Caissie et al., 2005). Most courses in special education or rehabilitative audiology teach students how to communicate with hearing-impaired children and adults. Some universities, clinics, and community health centers offer similar training to parents and family members. A traditional training course for communication partners typically includes information, instruction, observation, and participation.

Information

Most training courses include a review of important principles, such as those presented in the list below (McCall 1991; Erber 1993; Tye-Murray & Schum 1994). Awareness of principles alone, however, is not sufficient to ensure their regular use, and so further practical instruction is usually provided.

Principles for communicating with a hearing-impaired child

- ensure that an appropriate listening system is used
- speak at a short distance
- speak at the child's level
- speak slowly and carefully
- be sure your face is visible
- avoid environmental distractions
- relate messages to the situation and context

- match messages to the child's language level
- use common words in short, simple sentences
- indicate (changes of) topic
- pause between important thoughts
- allow time for the child to respond
- apply appropriate repair strategies
- check comprehension frequently

Instruction

Simply directing adults to speak more clearly can increase speech intelligibility for hearing-impaired listeners by approximately 10 to 30 per cent (Picheny et al., 1985; Gagné et al., 1994; Payton et al., 1994; Schum 1996; Bradlow et al., 2003). Similar guidance has been shown to produce an improvement of 8 per cent in *visual* intelligibility (Stoker & French-St. George 1987). Research suggests that even larger increases and longer-lasting improvement can be obtained through specific *instruction* (Caissie et al., 2005).

Instruction, observation, practice, and feedback are commonly used to improve the communication skills of newsreaders, actors, and other professional speakers. Similarly, an experienced teacher or therapist can instruct a parent in how to produce clear speech through more precise articulation, regular pauses, slower rate, and other strategies.

Observation

An adult can learn good communication practices by observing an experienced teacher interacting with a hearing-impaired child. This can occur incidentally (a parent observes a teacher speaking with her child's kindergarten group) or intentionally (a parent watches a video demonstration of specific communication strategies). These types of observation can be provided to family members and other communication partners at a weekend workshop.

Participation

It is common for university students to obtain practical experience in a classroom or clinic under the supervision of an experienced teacher or therapist before they attempt independent teaching or therapy. After each session, the supervisor and the student discuss the experience, and the instructor provides feedback. Parents of a young hearing-impaired child may be given similar opportunities to communicate with their child under the guidance of an experienced therapist.

A parent might also gain additional experience by working as a teacher's aide while the child attends pre-school, kindergarten, or school.

SIMULATION OF IMPAIRED HEARING

The traditional training methods described above are limited by:
- the adult's inability to understand the child's auditory experience
- the child's inability to provide useful feedback to the adult.

Ideally, parents, teachers, and therapists should develop effective communication skills without relying on the child for feedback.

In general, the quality of sound received by a hearing-impaired child is characterized by three main factors, even when the child listens through hearing aids or cochlear implants: (1) reduced sensitivity to sound, (2) different sound sensitivity at different frequencies, and (3) reduced clarity. Special electronic devices and computer software have been created to simulate the sound qualities of various types of hearing loss so that a person with normal hearing can hear what a hearing-impaired child hears (e.g., Gagné & Erber 1987; Nejime & Moore 1997; Howard-Jones et al., 2001; Erber 1995, 2008). For example, HELOS (Hearing Loss Simulator) software (Erber 2008) can produce a range of hearing thresholds, audiogram shapes, and auditory distortion effects including:
- an elevated hearing threshold (inability to hear low-intensity sounds)
- a sloping audiogram (poorer sensitivity at high frequencies)
- distortion (inability to hear audible speech sounds clearly).

By adjusting these three auditory effects, speech intelligibility can be varied from 0 to 100 per cent (Gagné & Erber 1987; Erber 1995, 2008). For many demonstrations and communication training, HELOS has been set to produce: an "aided" audiogram with thresholds of about 30 dB HL; a gradual downward slope above about 3000 Hz; and distortion that produces about 25 per cent auditory identification of one-syllable words.

In some cases, vision impairment has also been simulated with rough-surfaced (clear) plastic that is placed in front of a video camera lens or television screen (Erber 1979a; Erber & Yelland 1998). This can be calibrated by viewing a vision test chart (e.g., Snellen letters) through the video system. Visual acuity of approximately 6/120 (20/400) for Snellen test letters will generally impair perception of an adult's mouth movements at a conversational distance.

Educators have used hearing-loss simulation to produce audio and video recordings that simulate the auditory experiences of hearing-impaired children (Power 1991; Berlin 2007). Some recordings present a list of spoken words or sentences with reduced clarity to demonstrate the effects of impaired hearing on speech perception. Others depict a home or school environment from the child's point of view, to demonstrate effects of hearing impairment on daily communication.

Many parents, teachers, and university students have been introduced to the perceptual effects of hearing impairment in this way. The adult watches and listens to a video recording, learns how a hearing-impaired child might perceive speech, and gains empathy and insight into the child's daily life. This experience often stimulates the adult to think about ways to help the child communicate.

TRAINING WITH A HEARING-LOSS SIMULATOR

Hearing-loss simulation has been used for many years to train parents of hearing-impaired children, teachers, university students, and health professionals (Erber 2008). Most of these training procedures are interactive, incorporating role-play, observation, and communication practice with feedback. The participants learn how to produce clear speech and language, and how to apply clarification strategies. The main aims are (Erber 1996, 2002, 2008; Howard-Jones et al., 2001):

- to enable an adult to experience what a child hears
- to help the adult increase speech clarity, intelligibility, and conversational fluency
- to help the adult become a confident communication partner.

Communication training with a hearing-loss simulator typically includes:

- providing information about hearing loss and communication including principles of clear speech and language, and context and redundancy in spoken messages
- experience listening to speech and also communicating through a hearing-loss simulator
- proactive/reactive clarification strategies
- specific communication training activities
- observation and note-taking
- discussion of learning, strategies, personal progress
- self-assessment of knowledge, performance, confidence.

Information about hearing loss and communication

Most adults require some background information before they are ready to participate in communication training with a hearing-loss simulator. This information may include:

- types and degrees of hearing impairment
- the effects of impaired hearing on a child's ability to learn spoken language

- current methods of education/therapy
- how impaired hearing is simulated
- the benefits of clear speech and language on intelligibility
- appropriate communication strategies
- how to provide consistent feedback.

Principles of clear speech and language

Participants learn a variety of auditory and visual strategies to increase their speech and language clarity (Erber & Greer 1973; Erber 1982, 1985, 1993; Tye-Murray & Schum 1994) (see the following lists for *acoustic* and *visible* cues).

Some ways to enhance *acoustic* cues for speech

- maintain an adequate voice level
- maintain a stable voice pitch (avoid high pitch and large pitch shifts)
- articulate all speech sounds precisely
- increase the duration of vowels and continuant consonants
- emphasize articulatory contrast to clarify diphthongs, such as /eI, aI/
- provide emphasis to normally unstressed syllables
- speak more slowly than usual
- pause before and after key syllables, words, or phrases

Some ways to enhance *visible* cues for speech

- increase the duration of /m, n/ to distinguish these consonants from /p, b/ and /t, d/
- place the tongue between the upper and lower teeth to clarify the consonants /θ, ð/
- spread the lips and clench the teeth to indicate /s, z/
- bite the lower lip with the upper teeth to indicate /f, v/
- move the jaw downward briefly while producing /k, g/
- shrug the shoulders briefly during the inspiration preceding /h/
- increase or decrease the height/width of the lip aperture while producing extreme vowels, e.g., /i, ɑ, u/
- increase the duration of central vowels, such as /ʌ/
- emphasize articulatory contrast to clarify diphthongs, such as /eI, aI/
- speak a little more slowly than usual
- pause before and after key syllables, words, or phrases

Context and redundancy in spoken messages

Conversation does not occur in isolation. When people talk, they usually have a reason – something has happened, is happening, or is about to happen. *Context* refers to the setting or situation in which people communicate, and provides clues to what a person may be talking about or referring to (e.g., while eating breakfast, you might "slice bread/pour milk/eat cereal/drink coffee"). *Redundancy* refers to predictability within a particular phrase, sentence, or narrative resulting from meaningful relationships or rules of word order. Redundancy helps a listener anticipate what might come next (e.g., "She turned the key in the ____."). Both context and redundancy are major contributors to successful communication under difficult listening conditions.

Word-X

Some interactive "games" have been developed to help parents provide meaningful context and redundancy when they speak to their hearing-impaired child (Erber 1996, 2002, 2008). Parents generally participate in these activities *before* they practice communicating through a hearing-loss simulator. This builds familiarity with the application of proactive and reactive strategies.

Word-X is an interactive "game" in which a parent learns to speak words in meaningful contexts with speed and flexibility (Erber 1996, 2008). Two decks of shuffled cards are placed face down in front of the parent. Deck 1 contains cards printed with common target words (e.g., *book, apple, woman*). Deck 2 contains cards printed with one of three common contexts: "word" (related word), "sentence" (redundant sentence), or "story" (cohesive narrative). Another person plays the role of the hearing-impaired child. When this person says "Go!" and starts a countdown timer (e.g., set to 30 seconds), the parent picks up a card from each deck and attempts to communicate the target word by presenting it in the specified context (see figure 9.1). The parent is not permitted to say the target word, however, but must substitute the sound "bzzz" instead. The parent may present many different examples of the specified context. The "child" attempts to identify the word before the time period expires and the timer rings.

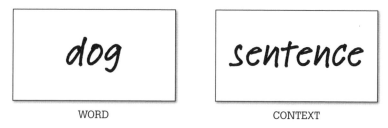

WORD   CONTEXT

Figure 9.1 **A word card ("dog") and a context card ("sentence") (Erber 2008)**

For example, if Word X is *dog*, an adult might provide the following contexts:

- Word context: "woof – bzzz"; "kennel – bzzz"; "greyhound – bzzz"
- Sentence context: "A poodle is a bzzz"; "A bzzz is man's best friend."
- Narrative context: "Sophie sleeps on a purple cushion. She jumps up and barks when someone comes to the door. Sophie is a bzzz."

LISTENING AND COMMUNICATION EXPERIENCE

A parent can learn effective communication skills, not only by *listening* through a hearing-loss simulator, but also by *interacting* with someone who simulates the child's hearing impairment.

To apply this approach, two participants must be positioned so that neither can hear the other directly. They may sit on opposite sides of a clear (not silvered) glass window in a hearing-test/observation room, or on opposite sides of a glass door or a door with a window that separates two rooms (see figure 9.2a). A double-glazed window is preferred, to minimize sound transmission. In another approach (Erber 1995, 1996), the participants sit in neighboring rooms, and communicate through a closed-circuit audio and video system (see figure 9.2b).

A microphone and pre-amplifier are used to deliver the parent's speech to HELOS. The parent's speech is modified by HELOS and delivered to a second person who plays the role of the hearing-impaired child. The "child" listens to modified speech and may also watch the parent for visible cues. The "child" uses a simple audio talkback system to describe which parts of the spoken message were understood, and to suggest strategies for increasing clarity. Parents clarify their speech and language as necessary to communicate successfully with the "child".

The participants can engage in many different communication activities. The parent may simply speak words (e.g., "cat", "bottle", "playground"), phrases (e.g., "four ripe tomatoes"), sentences (e.g., "My car has a flat tire"), or narrative (e.g., the contents of a brief newspaper article). In each case, the "child" attempts to understand and provides feedback. At other times, the two participants may engage in brief conversations (e.g., two to five minutes). Conversational topics may be selected at random from a list: e.g., travel, food, pets (Erber 2008).

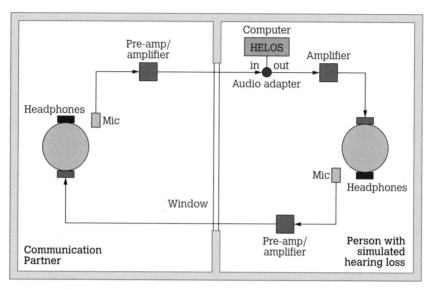

Figure 9.2a **Communication through a window (Erber 2008)**

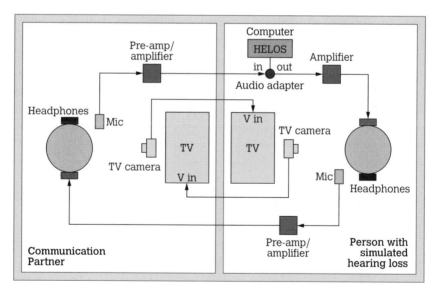

Figure 9.2b **Communication between two rooms (Erber 2008)**

Typically, participants work together during practice sessions distributed over many weeks, and may experience a variety of hearing (and vision) impairments. After training, their ability to apply communication strategies in real life is surveyed through discussion and a self-assessment questionnaire.

PROACTIVE/REACTIVE CLARIFICATION STRATEGIES

Early in training, most parents rely on the other person (the "child") for feedback regarding sources of difficulty and appropriate clarification strategies. For example, if articulation is imprecise or voice pitch is too high, the parent is asked to clarify. If a sentence is too complex, the parent is asked to simplify the message. If the context is insufficient, the parent is asked to provide more information.

As a result of practice with feedback, most parents learn to speak clearly and simply and to *anticipate* and thus prevent communication difficulties. A parent will generally pass through three stages while acquiring communication skills: (1) the parent relies on feedback, direction, and prompting from the person playing the role of the hearing-impaired child, (2) responsibility gradually shifts from the "child" to the parent, and (3) the parent communicates successfully without prompting.

High conversational fluency with a hearing-impaired child generally depends on the adult's successful use of *proactive* strategies. If the adult can avoid conversational breakdowns by communicating clearly, or can recognize difficulty and clarify spontaneously, the child will rarely need to request clarification, and conversational fluency will remain high. Stated simply, the best overall communication strategy is to avoid breakdowns in conversation.

COMMUNICATION-TRAINING ACTIVITIES

A wide variety of communication-training activities have been used with groups of parents and university students (Erber 1996, 2002, 2008). The following examples are meant as a guide only – the possibilities are almost limitless!

Vowel and consonant clarity

Some adults need practice in producing vowels and consonants with clear sound qualities or distinct mouth shapes for optimal intelligibility. Sets of vowels (spoken in /b/-vowel-/b/ sequence) and consonants (spoken in /ɑ/-consonant-/ɑ/ sequence) could be used for this purpose. When the parent presents each item through HELOS, the "child" listens and repeats what was perceived. Responses can be recorded on a stimulus-response diagram (matrix) for examination of error patterns (see Gagné & Erber 1987). Later, specific practice can be directed to correcting persistent deviations in articulation.

Communicating common words with specific feedback and guidance

In this activity, a parent learns many ways to enhance word intelligibility. Parents often collect lists of common words that their hearing-impaired child persistently misunderstands. They usually want to know (1) why these items are so hard to communicate and (2) how to make them intelligible. Words may be combined to form a general vocabulary list, or they may be separated into categories: for example, clothing, furniture, transportation, people, or food. Alternatively, a published list of common words can be used (Erber 2008) (see Appendix 3).

Each word is written on a separate card, the deck is shuffled, and 20 cards are placed in front of the parent (printed side down). The parent turns over a card and attempts to communicate the word to the "child" who listens through HELOS. The "child" repeats whatever was received (even nonsense). If the "child" identifies the word correctly, the parent proceeds to the next card and speaks the next word. If the response is not correct, the "child" analyzes the difficulty and suggests specific strategies, such as "say it again", "talk more slowly", "say the word in a sentence."

The parent increases clarity and provides context as requested. Several different strategies may be required to communicate the word successfully. When the "child" eventually identifies the word, the parent may proceed to the next one. When all word-cards are completed, the two participants exchange roles. For example (word = elbow):

- elbow >> lawn mower ... but I know that's wrong. Please say it in a sentence.
- The elbow is part of my arm. >> lawn mower on the farm? Try a different sentence.
- I bumped my elbow on the table. >> I bumped my elbow on the table – elbow!

Further examples of common words and communication strategies that have led to their identification include:

- bed – sentence: "It's time for bed!"
- puzzle – phrase: "a piece of the jigsaw puzzle"
- curtain – sentence: "The curtain is on the window."
- carpet – related word: vacuum cleaner > carpet
- pin – sentence: "The pin is very sharp!"
- nappy – sentence: "The baby wears a nappy."
- color – sentence: "Purple is a color."
- nose – related words: mouth, eyes ... nose
- comb – sentence: "Comb your hair."
- tooth – emphasized last speech sound /θ/
- hair – sentence: "Wash your hair."

- sugar – emphasized first speech sound /ʃ/
- bird – sentence: "The bird flew into the big tree."
- cupboard – sentence: "Put the dishes in the cupboard."
- fork – related words: spoon, knife … fork.
- cheese – sentence: "Would you like to eat some cheese?"
- cake – related word: birthday … cake
- circle – sentence: "Draw a circle on the paper."
- shampoo – stressed last syllable: sham<u>poo</u>
- garden – related words: flower, tree … garden.

Communicating words without specific feedback or guidance

In this practice activity, parents learn how to communicate words clearly and apply contextual strategies *without* specific feedback or guidance from the "child" (Erber 2008). This is important because young hearing-impaired children generally lack the skills required to provide specific feedback regarding the intelligibility of their parents' speech, or to suggest appropriate clarification strategies.

Twenty word-cards (randomly selected from a large set) are placed in front of the parent (printed side down). The parent takes the top card and speaks the word through HELOS to the "child". The "child" is not permitted to repeat any part of the message, but must simply respond with either "yes" (I am 90+ per cent confident that I know what you said) or "no" (I am not 90+ per cent confident that I know what you said).

If the "child" responds "yes", the parent proceeds to the next word-card. If the "child" responds "no", the *parent* must analyze the difficulty, and apply appropriate clarification strategies. This is a closer approximation to real life, where the parent must make the necessary adjustments without specific instruction or guidance from the child. The parent may need to apply several different strategies to communicate successfully.

Each time the "child" responds "yes" (i.e., word-identification with confidence), he/she should write down what was perceived. Later, the "child" compares this written list with the set of words that were actually spoken. Then the two participants exchange roles. For example:

- Word: hamburger >> yes (writes "hamburger" – this is correct)
- Word: table >> yes (writes "staple" – this is incorrect and will require discussion on completion of the activity)
- Word: scissors >> no
  s c i s s o r s (slower) >> no
  rock, paper, scissors (phrase) >> no
  I cut a piece of paper with my scissors. (sentence) >> yes (writes "scissors" – this is correct)

Identifying "easy" and "difficult" words

This activity is another variation on those described above. After communicating a word, the parent places the card in either an EASY or DIFFICULT pile according to the number of clarification attempts required (see table 9.1). The parent examines the words in each pile and considers both common and differing features. Later, the parent receives a new set of cards and attempts to predict which words will be easy/difficult to communicate *before* speaking them. The parent and the instructor may also discuss potential sources of difficulty; for example, the number of syllables in a word, acoustic similarities between words, and visual similarities between words (Kirk et al., 1995).

Table 9.1 **A mother spoke common words through HELOS to a therapist who played the role of her child. The mother judged each word as EASY or DIFFICULT to communicate**

EASY		DIFFICULT
grandpa	nail	watch
bedroom	basket	shower
grandma	wood	block
train	grass	scissors
glass	bed	bike
bedroom	sausage	sheep
birthday	name	shirt
water	blanket	bin
butter	tummy	cat
shelf	food	tree
washer	bear	mess
bath	nanna	shoe
window	wheel	nappy
banana	ball	fridge
balloon	truck	bird
sandpit	bathroom	feet
14 one-syllable words		13 one-syllable words
17 two-syllable words		3 two-syllable words
1 three-syllable word		0 three-syllable words

Communicating phrases and sentences

In general, when adults speak to hearing-impaired children, they express themselves through phrases and sentences. Phrases are short samples of spoken language that contain several key elements and illustrate syntactic/semantic relationships (Montgomery & Houston 2000). Common types include prepositional phrases ("in the big box"), adjective-noun phrases ("brown bear"), or noun phrases like those in a shopping list ("four litres of apple juice") (Erber 2008).

Types of sentences may include descriptions ("Jan has a new red and white dress!"), opinions ("I think your hair is beautiful!"), feelings ("I'm very angry!"), or questions. Questions range from those that limit possible responses ("Do you want orange or apple juice?") to less restrictive types ("Where is the broom?") and open questions ("What kind of games do you like?").

Parents and teachers can prepare lists of phrases and sentences for presentation during HELOS communication practice. An interactive procedure, such as QUEST?AR (see pp. 88–90, or A:SQUE (see pp. 124–5) also might be used as a source of questions and statements (Erber 1996).

Regardless of the practice material, a similar procedure is followed. The instructor writes each phrase or sentence on a card, places the cards in a deck, shuffles and stacks them in front of the parent (printed side down). The parent turns over the top card and speaks the phrase or sentence through HELOS. The "child" listens, watches carefully, and repeats. If correct, the participants proceed to the next item. If difficulty occurs, however, the "child" suggests strategies to increase understanding. The activity can then be repeated without specific feedback or clarification, and in a natural conversational style.

In most of these communication-training activities, each participant plays two roles: (1) a hearing-impaired "child", who listens to speech under difficult perceptual conditions, and (2) an adult who must communicate effectively to overcome the effects of these listening conditions. Thus, a participant has two complementary learning objectives: (1) to learn how hearing impairment can *reduce* the fluency of conversation, and (2) to learn how to select and use communication strategies to *increase* the fluency of conversation (Erber & Lind 1994; Howard-Jones et al., 2001).

Transcribing sentences

In this practice activity, the parent speaks sentences through HELOS to the "child", who speaks and also writes down what is perceived (including fragments or nonsense), but is *not* permitted to guide the parent. The parent considers the errors and selects a repair strategy. The parent is permitted to present each sentence up to five times (Erber 2008).

Written transcriptions (see the list below) show sequences of auditory errors which lead to correct identification. In some cases, the most important part of a sentence (e.g., a noun phrase or verb phrase) is not identified first, especially if it contains a rare word, an unclear mouth movement, or a weak syllable.

Responses to repeated presentation of sentences through HELOS

The na fine number.
There the sanke is very hot.
You namontel looks nice.
Your _____ is a monkey.
Your appointment is on Monday. (unexpected word)

This is the Queen of England.
This is a safe haven.
Take out the _____ of the oven.
_____ the cake out of the oven.
She took the cake out of the oven. (high frequency sounds)

___ ___ ___ ___ ___ ___ ___ ___ (8 syllables?)
_____ uh eh _____aye _____ ing _____
_____ girl doesn't eat a three.
That _____ doesn't fit very well.
That shirt doesn't fit very well. (inanimate subject)

Conversation through a hearing-loss simulator

Most daily interaction occurs as face-to-face conversation. In a realistic communication activity, participants select topics from a deck of topic cards (Erber 2008) and engage in brief conversations through HELOS (e.g., two to five minutes). They imagine familiar situations and play appropriate roles. Bluffing is not permitted, so when a misunderstanding occurs, clarification is required before the conversation can proceed: (1) the parent may spontaneously clarify, (2) the "child" may request a particular strategy (e.g., talk louder; speak slower; simplify) or (3) the instructor may recommend a type of clarification.

Following each conversation, the participants rate conversational fluency on a scale from 1 (low) to 4 (high) as shown in table 5.2 (Erber 1996, 2002, 2008). The participants discuss how the hearing impairment and specific conversational strategies influenced the flow of conversation.

Conversational strategies that speech-language therapy students found to be effective during this activity are listed below. These strategies included slowed speech, clear speech, repetition, and short sentences containing familiar words (Erber 1996).

Effective strategies used by student therapists during conversations through HELOS (Erber 1996)

- speak slowly
- discuss familiar aspects of the topic
- articulate clearly
- repeat a word, phrase, or sentence
- use uncomplicated syntax
- speak predictable words, phrases, and sentences
- comply with specific requests for clarification
- speak short sentences
- present associated word(s)
- rephrase sentences
- maintain topic
- use common words

OBSERVATION AND NOTE-TAKING

If a group of learners contains more than two people, the extra participants may observe and write notes. An observer might record:

- HELOS settings
- each item that was spoken by the adult
- the "child's" responses
- the sequence of clarification strategies
- the final (successful) strategy
- the amount of effort that was required
- words that were difficult to identify (e.g., *cake*)
- the sequence of strategies that lead to correct identification
- effective prompts (e.g., "birthday > cake").
- parts of sentences that were inaudible (e.g., the last word)
- particular mouth movements that were invisible (e.g., initial /k/)
- confusing mouth movements (e.g., speaker bites lower lip when pausing)
- words/phrases that were confused with one another (e.g., "it is" – "is it")
- particular words/phrases/sentences that were very easy to identify (e.g., *popcorn*) or very difficult (e.g., *kitchen*)
- voice qualities (e.g., high pitch) or mouth movements (e.g., the consonant blend in *clap*) that were sources of difficulty.

GROUP DISCUSSION

Group discussion is an important part of each training session. During this time, participants discuss practice material that was easy or difficult to communicate, and clarification strategies that were effective or ineffective in particular circumstances. They may also discuss how they have modified their everyday speech and language as a result of experience gained while communicating through HELOS.

SELF-ASSESSMENT QUESTIONNAIRE

After training, participants also complete a brief questionnaire in which they are asked to describe:
- their own speech and language characteristics
- changes in their speech and language after training
- what they learned from the child's point of view
- general benefits of role-play
- carryover of learning into communication at home.

Awareness of own speech/language

Comments from previous participants (parents) include:
- I was surprised that words are so different in intelligibility.
- My voice is sometimes too soft during small words and toward the end of a sentence.
- I didn't realize that a child might hear something so different from what I heard myself say.
- I discovered that I had been running my words together, not pausing to indicate syllables and word separation.
- My voice pitch is often a little too high.
- I need to practice speaking simpler sentences. Some are too long for a child to absorb all the information. I need to break a sentence into smaller parts that can be understood.
- I didn't realize that I speak with a loud voice! Maybe this is good for my daughter though – it makes it easier to hear me!

Changes to own speech/language

Comments from previous participants (parents) include:
- I learned to speak more slowly and pause before key words.
- I'm learning to pronounce words more clearly.

- I realized it's important to make my face visible and in a good light.
- I learned to say the sounds in each word carefully – especially consonant blends – because the second sound tends to disappear unless I say it carefully.
- I've learned how to choose words that are easier to understand.
- I discovered that intonation often adds to the meaning of a sentence.
- I didn't realize that I moved my head so much when I talked.
- I found that slightly slowing and slightly exaggerating my speech has increased my intelligibility.
- I found that rephrasing with extra information helps.
- I've become very aware of the importance of keeping my voice level as I talk.
- I'm learning how to structure sentences to make them easier to understand.
- I need to avoid vague language: rather than say "Put it there!" I should say "Put the cup on the table!"

The child's point of view

Comments from previous participants (parents) include:
- I learned that my daughter needs a lot more information than she's been getting from me. It is a lot harder than I imagined!
- I was surprised at the order in which I identified words in sentences.
- I learned that the expression on a person's face conveys a lot of information.
- At first, the speech sounded very strange. After a while, I became aware of the syllables and rhythm.
- I found that visibility of a person's mouth movements can help make sense of a partly heard sentence.
- I didn't realize it could be so hard to hear the word "milk"! "Chocolate milk" is much easier!
- I realized that voiceless consonants are much less audible unless a person says them carefully.
- I didn't realize how much a hearing-impaired child needs to concentrate to understand what someone is saying.
- I found that people's voice levels were very different. With some speakers, I was only able to hear a few vowels in a sentence.
- I found that a visible mouth pattern sometimes helped me decide between two similar words that sounded alike.

Role-playing

Comments from previous participants (parents) include:
- Role–playing helped me relate the practice activities to everyday experiences with my child.
- It was important to have a turn as both talker and listener.

- The context of a situation was important for understanding.
- It was useful and interesting learning how to communicate statements and questions that I actually use every day.

Follow-up at home

Comments from previous participants (parents) include:
- I told my husband about the strategies that worked best for me. He tried some of them and found that they helped.
- Communication practice gave me confidence as a speaker. My daughter responds to me much better now and is more willing than ever before to repeat sounds and try new words.
- My husband and I talk about the words that have been hard for me to communicate.
- I told my husband to communicate at the same level, make eye contact, speak a little louder, and be willing to repeat. He's stopped talking in only one- or two-word sentences, and is beginning to use the same strategies when he talks to our other child (who has normal hearing)! He's been very surprised with the positive responses received from our daughter (who has a hearing impairment).
- I've become much more aware of our son's needs when talking with him at home.
- I explained the program to my husband and passed on the information, but I don't like telling him how he should interact with Jackie. I feel that he would benefit from doing the communication course himself.

ORGANIZATION OF PRACTICE SESSIONS

Although it is possible to introduce hearing-loss simulation to a large group of parents, teachers, or therapists in the form of a short course, it is recommended that you create *small* groups for regular (e.g., weekly) communication practice, for approximately four to eight weeks. A convenient group size is about two to four participants, plus an instructor who plans, participates in, and facilitates the sessions.

Participants will sometimes play the role of the "adult" and practice producing clear speech and language. At other times, they will play the role of the hearing-impaired "child" and provide feedback and guidance.

A typical weekly session might be organized as follows:
- the instructor reviews previous activities
- each participant describes recent real-life communication experiences
- the instructor describes the current day's activities
- each pair communicates through HELOS for about 15 to 20 minutes
- the "adult" and "child" exchange roles

- the instructor facilitates discussion of communication difficulties and effective strategies
- the instructor assigns home activities – e.g., "Apply what you learned in this session to real conversations with your child."

SUMMARY

This chapter has described how you can use HELOS hearing-loss simulation software to provide live interactive experience to parents, teachers, and students. During training, each participant plays two roles: (1) an adult communicator, and (2) a child with impaired hearing. Each participant learns effective communication strategies through demonstrations and practical activities.

Training with a hearing-loss simulator enables communication partners of hearing-impaired children to:
- gain insight into the child's auditory experience
- converse under different conditions of sensory loss
- learn to speak clearly and simply
- learn how to avoid communication difficulties
- learn how to resolve communication difficulties
- experience success as a communicator.

CHAPTER 10

Review and conclusion

A young hearing-impaired child learns to listen and communicate through a complex process – one that relies on many factors for success. This chapter briefly reviews the key components of the auditory communication process, and describes strategies that can facilitate a child's auditory learning.

AUDITORY COMMUNICATION PROCESS

The main components of the auditory communication process are:

1 *What you say* – you formulate a message that is related to the situation, activity, and/or conversational context.
2 *How you say it* – vocal sounds generated by your larynx are altered by your lips, tongue and other articulators to produce speech. You monitor your own speech clarity, and by listening while speaking.
3 *The environment* – your speech travels through the acoustic environment on its way to the child. Noise and echo may affect the clarity of your spoken message.
4 *Personal listening system* – the sounds of your speech also pass through the child's hearing aids or cochlear implants. Some speech qualities are made more or less prominent than others.
5 *Detection of speech* – the child's auditory system receives your speech after it is modified by hearing aids or cochlear implants. Each sound stimulus produces nerve impulses that are conveyed to the child's brain.
6 *Discrimination, identification, comprehension* – the child's brain interprets the nerve impulses on the basis of previously acquired experience and linguistic processes.
7 *Child's response* – the behavioral or spoken response indicates whether the child received your spoken message as you intended.
8 *Adult's adaptive behavior* – if the child received your message correctly, you are likely to speak another related message. If, however, the child did not understand what you said, then you may repeat, clarify, modify the message, or provide additional information.

WHAT YOU SAY

A child's ability to perceive a spoken message is affected by its structure and content. Sentences are generally easier to identify if they are linguistically simple (or at least matched to the child's language level) and if they contain speech sounds, words, or phrases that are acoustically distinctive (Kirk et al., 1995). Message perception can be improved by orienting the child to the conversation topic, using simple word order, and increasing redundancy. A hearing-impaired child is also more likely to understand a spoken message if it is part of the current activity and occurs at an appropriate point in the conversation.

A hearing-impaired child can learn to use context to identify a mis-heard speech sound, word, or sentence. For example, through play in the bath, a child may learn to associate the unclear sound quality /boUp/ ("bope") with his toy boat. Later, through play with toy farm animals, the child may hear another speech pattern (the spoken word *goat*) that sounds essentially the same: "bope". An adult can help the child to use contextual information to identify which item has been spoken (see Nittrouer & Boothroyd 1990; Olsen et al., 1997). If the child's mother fills the bathtub, and the child hears her say, "It's time for your bath … where's your bope?" the child may presume that she said the word *boat*. If his pre-school teacher points to a picture in a book, and the child hears her say, "The bope ate all the farmer's strawberries!" the child may reasonably conclude that she said the word *goat*.

HOW YOU SAY IT

Speech clarity is a function of the sound qualities produced by the speaker's larynx and the movements of the lips, tongue, and other articulators. Factors that can reduce speech clarity include high voice pitch, low intensity, rapid rate, and imprecise articulation.

An adult's speech intelligibility can be improved through training (Gagné et al., 1994; Caissie et al., 2005). In general, clear speech is characterized by a slow speech rate, slightly increased intensity, careful articulation, and moderate emphasis on each syllable (Uchanski 2005). You may benefit from using hearing loss simulation software (Erber 2008) to experiment with different speech intensities and rates to determine which produce the greatest intelligibility. You can also encourage the child to inform you if your speech is too loud, too soft, too fast, or distorted in some way.

THE ENVIRONMENT

The surroundings in which communication occurs can affect what the child hears. The acoustic conditions may not be ideal. For example, other people may be talking nearby, traffic noise may be audible, the room may echo, or other distractions may be present. Visual conditions, such as glare or poor lighting, also can disrupt communication. To ensure a smooth flow of conversation, the adult must be able to recognize and manage a poor communication environment. This requires vigilance, flexibility, and a repertoire of strategies.

Noise and echo

Children with impaired hearing need a quiet listening environment because noise and echo can seriously interfere with communication and learning (Erber & Zeiser 1974; Finitzo-Hieber & Tillman 1978; Ross 1992; Nelson & Soli 2000; Smaldino et al., 2008).

Parents and teachers can promote a good listening environment in the home or classroom by:

- using a wireless FM communication system consistently, where the microphone is close to the speaker's mouth
- regularly assessing ambient noise
- showing children how to monitor their own voice levels
- providing tasks to keep children busy and quiet
- closing doors and windows when possible to exclude noise
- reducing echo with soft furnishings, window coverings, and carpets/mats
- turning off noisy fans, air conditioners, computers, and data projectors when possible
- showing the hearing-impaired child how to find the best place for good communication (not near a fan/air conditioner duct)
- using an appropriate voice level that the child can hear and understand
- checking listening and comprehension regularly (e.g., "Danny, what did Sarah say?").

Listening in noise

The goal of an early intervention program is to prepare a hearing-impaired child for a lifetime of auditory communication. Adults interact with the child in quiet to make listening and learning easier. These early experiences, however, may not prepare a child for auditory communication in a noisy pre-school or classroom, where listening and learning are more complex and tiring. Listening practice in a moderately distracting environment may be beneficial, where the amount of background noise is gradually increased over a long period of time.

Illumination

A child with impaired hearing may frequently rely on visual cues for communication. The optical (visible) environment can impair a child's ability to perceive speech through lipreading (Erber & Zeiser 1974). A viewing angle beyond approximately 45 degrees and a viewing distance greater than a few meters can reduce lipreading performance (Erber 1971, 1974a). Reflections and extreme brightness contrasts also may cause visual difficulty. Ideally you should avoid standing in front of a window on a sunny day, or standing in front of distracting activities. Try to face the main source of light and try to keep the conversational distance short.

THE CHILD'S PERSONAL LISTENING SYSTEM

It is primarily an adult's responsibility to ensure that the sounds of speech are delivered clearly and reliably to a young child through an appropriate listening system. Optimal programming/mapping of a child's hearing aids or cochlear implants is a crucial factor in ensuring auditory learning. It is important to create daily routines for testing and maintenance of hearing aids, cochlear implants, and/or FM system. It is also important to teach the child relevant vocabulary and language to describe your speech quality (e.g., "Your voice is clear and you are close. That's my FM sound" or "Your voice is far away, and mixed up with noise.")

THE CHILD'S HEARING

The child's auditory system receives your speech after it has been modified by hearing aids or cochlear implants. Sound is converted into nerve impulses that are conveyed to the brain. The child's brain interprets the patterns of nerve impulses through linguistic processes based on life experiences. Auditory learning occurs when you speak in meaningful situations, respond to the child in timely and appropriate ways, and link current skills to more complex auditory tasks.

A child's ability to perceive speech can decrease as a result of fatigue, reduced attention, middle-ear disease, and/or poor health. Irritation of the outer ear (pinna, ear canal) can reduce a child's use of any listening device worn on or in the ear (e.g., an earmold, hearing aid, or implant processor). If speech perception ability is decreased, this can impair auditory learning. Routinely examine the child's ears and observe auditory behavior. Administer a simple speech-detection test daily to monitor the child's hearing (e.g., the Ling 6-sound test). The child should be referred to an audiologist and/or doctor if you observe any change.

THE CHILD'S VISION

Vision impairment is common among children with impaired hearing, ranging between 30 and 60 per cent of children in special classes (Levin & Erber 1976; Armitage et al., 1995). Some vision disorders can cause a significant reduction in lipreading performance (Karp 1988).

It is therefore important to be alert for signs of vision impairment such as a deviant eye, squinting, visual fatigue, or frequent headaches, all of which require referral to a pediatric eye specialist. For children who use eyeglasses for vision correction, check for dirty/scratched lenses or loose/bent frames that could interfere with visual (and thus auditory-visual) perception. In cases where a child has an uncorrectable vision disorder, such as reduced visual fields or color blindness, adaptations may be beneficial such as optimal seating, good illumination, large print, high contrast, and appropriate colors on learning materials.

THE CHILD'S RESPONSE

The response to your spoken message usually indicates whether or not the child has understood what you said. Possible responses include:

- confused facial expression – suggesting that the child understood little of the message
- long silence or apparent bluffing – the child is unsure whether the message was received correctly. You may wish to investigate with questions such as: "What are you thinking?" or "What did you hear?"
- inappropriate response – e.g., when leaving the house, the parent asks "Have you got your hat?" but the child responds "Yes. She ate all her food." This response suggests that the child perceived the question as, "Have you fed the cat?"
- frequent misunderstandings – may suggest insufficient contextual information. You may wish to provide a supplementary cue, picture/diagram, or spoken prompt (e.g., "Remember when …?")
- abrupt topic shift – often a result of misunderstanding. You could verify that the child is following the flow of conversation and/or investigate the source of confusion (e.g., distraction, inattention, fatigue).

The child also has an important role to play in the management of conversation. The child should learn how to recognize common reasons for conversational difficulty (speech too fast, message too long, too much noise, communication partner too far away, listening system not working), and ask for appropriate help. You may wish to teach the child specific requests for clarification such as "Please don't talk so fast!" or "I can't hear you – the TV is too loud!"

THE ADULT'S ADAPTIVE BEHAVIOR

A hearing-impaired child's communicative progress depends on regular opportunities to experience *success* as a listener and communicator. An adult can maintain interest and motivation by letting the child choose the conversation topic and by using appropriate adaptive strategies to avoid and/or repair conversation breakdown. These strategies include:

- repetition – saying the message again
- clarification – greater intensity, slower rate, increased clarity
- phrase, sentence, or conversational context
- supplementary information – e.g., a related picture or object
- visible cues for mouth shapes and movements
- facial cues that convey emotion, meaning, or intent
- gestural cues such as pointing or miming.

CONCLUSION

This book has provided a practical approach to the development of auditory communication skills in a child with impaired hearing. One-to-one interaction with adults, such as parents, teachers, and therapists is highly recommended. It is important, however, that the child also has frequent opportunities for listening and communicating in small groups with other children, and a variety of other learning and play activities.

It is important to provide the child with a reasonable balance between *auditory-visual* communication to present important information and *auditory* experience to promote the development of listening skills. It is also important to be flexible and creative as you adapt activities to the child's needs, interests, and abilities.

Many factors influence auditory communication and learning. The following conditions will enable a child to experience success:

- a functioning personal listening system
- a good listening environment
- a meaningful situation
- interesting learning materials
- creative instructional methods
- audible and clear speech
- appropriate spoken language
- suitable adaptive strategies
- empathy and cooperation.

The principles and methods described throughout this book offer a practical framework for parents, teachers, and therapists who wish to provide auditory communication and learning opportunities for hearing-impaired children. If you apply these methods appropriately and creatively, you can help your child reach potential as an auditory communicator.

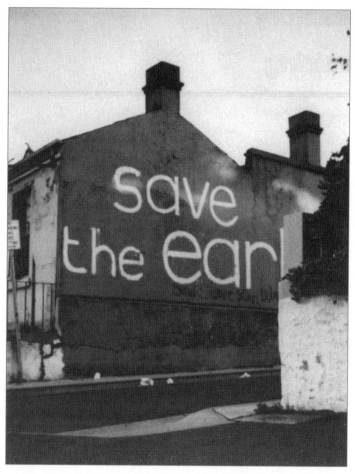

Graffiti on Lygon Street at the corner of Waterloo Street, Carlton (first published in Erber 1982).

APPENDIX 1

Notes for teachers

AUDITORY AND AUDITORY-VISUAL COMMUNICATION

Face-to-face interaction is an important part of a young child's social and emotional development, and most children learn to communicate through hearing and vision together (Locke 1993; Marshall & Fox 2006). In general, hearing-impaired children understand speech better when they lipread as they listen (Erber 1975; Lachs et al., 2001). Some communication experiences that contribute to a child's auditory-visual acquisition of spoken language include:

- a short distance between the adult and the child
- regular eye contact and mutual gaze
- using facial expressions to convey emotional states
- associating vocal output and facial expressions
- imitating vocal output and facial expressions.

When important information must be conveyed, combined auditory-visual communication is generally the best method. When the aim, however, is to develop the child's ability to perceive speech sounds and develop auditory communication skills, then practice attending to acoustic cues *alone* can be beneficial. If one of the aims is to enable telephone conversation without visible cues, the child *must* learn to receive spoken messages through listening alone.

Parents and therapists generally want to know whether to exclude visible cues during development of speech communication (a uni-sensory approach), or whether to allow the child to lipread while listening (a multi-sensory approach). Advocates for each approach claim that their preferred system is the most effective means for language development. Those who promote an auditory method believe that this approach provides the best opportunity to develop a language-processing system based on sound and hearing (Pollack et al., 1997). Those who favor a multi-sensory method believe that combining the speech information available through each sense will maximize language acquisition and social development (Simmons-Martin & Rossi 1990; Moog et al., 1994).

A direct comparison between uni-sensory and multi-sensory instruction is difficult, however, because exclusive application of each method is uncommon. Educators who recommend auditory-only procedures acknowledge that: (1) it is impractical for parents to exclude visible cues for speech all of the time, (2) some communication partners (e.g., the child's grandparents) might prefer face-to-face conversation and (3) many people on television are visible as they talk. On the other hand, auditory-visual advocates are unable to exclude auditory-only communication experiences such as: (1) when their faces are turned to speak to another child, (2) when driving a car and (3) when speaking at night in a dark place.

A balanced approach to auditory learning is probably the best strategy. This involves providing listening opportunities throughout the day and encouraging the child to listen to a part of everything you say. Observe the child's behavior, be flexible, and adapt appropriately. If listening without visible cues seems to interfere with communication and learning, and if this is too difficult/exhausting for the child, or affects social behavior, adopt a face-to-face approach as needed. When the child is experiencing success and seems confident, try speaking with your mouth obscured more often, and monitor the child's communication and learning by listening alone.

INDIVIDUAL AND GROUP INTERACTION

Most educators of young hearing-impaired children recommend one-to-one interaction because it allows an adult to give individual attention for long periods of time without interruption (Beebe 1953; Pollack 1970; Estabrooks 1994; Simser 1999). It also allows the adult to adapt topics and materials to the child's specific interests, abilities, and needs. It may be possible to reach listening goals more quickly with one-to-one interaction (Pollack 1984). When only one child is present, the surroundings are likely to be relatively quiet and free of distractions, and an adult's speech is heard more easily (see figure A1.1). During one-to-one interaction, it is usually easy to attract and maintain the child's attention. Close proximity also allows the adult to manipulate pictures or objects near the child, and guide responses.

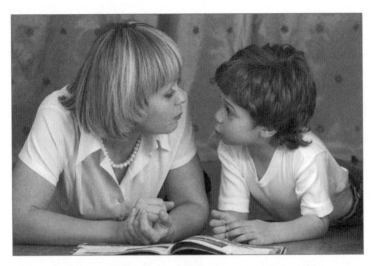

Figure A1.1 **One-to-one communication with a child**

In many schools and clinics, however, adults teach children in small groups (Moog 2002). Working in a *group* also has advantages. For example, a child learns how to behave socially, take turns in conversation, and cooperate with others. Participation in games and conversations with other children promotes social relationships with peers. Children usually develop listening and conversational skills in contexts that are meaningful to *children*. Small-group activities with other children provide opportunities for natural interaction, where appropriate communication skills are learned. In a group, children can help one another by offering prompts, strategies, or encouragement.

A hearing-impaired child often learns spoken language and self-help strategies from social interaction with children who have normal hearing. The hearing-impaired child will usually be motivated by other children and is likely to learn appropriate behavior quickly.

In practice, most teachers combine group and individual instruction, and try to arrange auditory experiences within small groups of two or three children. The teacher can then conduct either a group conversation or direct attention to an individual child.

CLASSROOM MANAGEMENT

Planning auditory experiences

In order to maximize each child's communication development, it is important to anticipate and plan appropriate auditory experiences. A basic lesson sequence might include:

1 Beginning with a brief *introductory* activity to orient the child to the task – something easy, such as naming the words that will be used (e.g., *corn, pumpkin, potato, asparagus*).

2 Presenting a *main* activity in which you try something that may be new or difficult. Take risks and challenge the child with unpracticed listening activities, such as remembering a sequence of three spoken instructions, or answering several comprehension questions after you have told a short story.

3 Concluding with a brief *departure* activity, such as presenting a familiar auditory task to sustain each child's confidence as a listener. For example, you might say, "Billy, it's time for lunch!" or "Belinda, pick up your books!" Always try to conclude with a listening task at which the child can succeed. The purpose is to maintain a positive attitude toward listening.

It is also important to be flexible and responsive to the child's behavior and feedback. If you discover that an activity you have prepared is too easy or too difficult, you should change the activity to suit the child's auditory skill level. For example, if you have planned a word-identification activity with pictures of farm animals, and it is too easy, ask comprehension questions about farm animals, wild animals, or household pets. If the task is too *difficult*, reduce the number of items in the set, include words with different stress patterns, or present a simpler listening task at the discrimination level.

Listening activities

Do not spend much time on lower-level auditory tasks (e.g., detection of speech sounds) if a child is capable of listening at a much higher level (e.g., identification or comprehension of sentences). Try to give the child the most practice at the highest possible level. Introduce higher-level tasks as a challenge. Use lower-level tasks mainly as remedial "investigative" activities when you are not sure why a child has failed to respond correctly. You also may introduce an easy listening activity as a change of pace during a difficult listening activity, or to allow the child to experience success without extreme effort.

Try to provide variety in listening activities, so that the child remains interested and alert. Relate each listening activity to a different theme such as "how to make a pizza", "growing vegetables", or "where spiders live".

Perception through a vibro-tactile system

A child with poor hearing may lack awareness of sound in the environment, or have difficulty perceiving rhythmic details in speech. The child may benefit from receiving "sound" through a tactile vibrator. Vibro-tactile systems have been used as part of communication training for many years (Gault 1927, 1930; Guberina 1964; Erber 1978; Schulte 1978; Osberger et al., 1991a, 1991b; Weisenberger & Percy 1994).

A simple vibro-tactile aid is constructed from a microphone, amplifier, and bone-conduction transducer (e.g., as used in bone-conduction hearing tests), and the child uses his/her fingertips to feel the output. A child can easily learn to feel and perceive changes in sound *intensity*, such as number of syllables or stress pattern. A more complex multi-channel vibro-tactile system might contain a speech processor and more than one tactile vibrator. Each vibrator could convey information about a limited range of speech frequencies or a specific speech feature (e.g., frication), and the child would feel each cue with a different finger, or part of the hand.

A child can use tactile cues to distinguish the patterns of words and sentences. Tactile cues for voicing, nasality, and frication can help the child to lipread some speech sounds that look alike (e.g., /f, v/). Tactile cues allow the child to monitor his/her own speech by providing an indication of loudness, rate, and rhythm. It is difficult for a child to learn to identify spoken words or the content of sentences tactually, unless visible cues are available, or the response choices are limited.

Vibro-tactile training is similar to auditory training, but with attention directed to the *intensity patterns* of speech. A recommended approach includes not only practicing (1) recognition of vibro-tactile qualities (e.g., duration, intensity, rate, roughness), but also (2) acquisition of meaning during face-to-face interaction (e.g., "They delivered 14 [or 40?] boxes of books.") (Plant 1994).

Words spoken to young children

This list of common nouns was contributed by a group of 20 pre-school teachers and parents of young hearing-impaired children. They reported that they spoke each of these words at least once per week, and some words were spoken frequently. You may select items from this list for use in listening activities.

animal	clock	ground	neck	sister
apple	clothes	hair	night	skirt
arm	coat	hammer	noise	sky
baby	coffee	hand	nose	snail
back	color	hankie	orange	spoon
bag	comb	hat	orange juice	soap
ball	computer	head	outside	sock
balloon	cook	hearing aid	oven	song
banana	cough	hole	page	soup
basket	cow	home	paint	sponge
bath	crayon	honey	pants	stairs
bathroom	cup	horse	paper	stone
bear	cupboard	house	paste	story
bed	curtain	ice-cream	peg	street
bedroom	daddy	jacket	pen	sugar
bike	dance	jam	pencil	sultana
bin	day	jeans	phone	sun
bird	dinner	jigsaw	photo	swing
birthday	dog	jumper	picture	table
biscuit	doll	juice	pig	tail
blanket	door	kangaroo	pin	tap
blocks	drawer	key	plane	tea

boat	drawing	kids	plant	teddy
book	dress	kindergarten	plate	tee-shirt
bottle	drink	kiss	pocket	teeth
bottom	drum	kitchen	pram	telephone
bowl	duck	knee	pusher	television
box	ear	knife	puzzle	thumb
boy	egg	lamb	rabbit	tin
bread	elephant	laundry	radio	tissue
breakfast	eye	leaf	rain	toast
broom	face	leg	ring	toe
brother	finger	letter	road	toilet
brush	fish	lid	rock	tongue
bubbles	floor	light	room	tooth
bucket	flower	lolly	rubbish	towel
bus	fly	lunch	rubbish bin	toy
butter	food	man	sand	tractor
button	foot	mat	sandpit	train
cake	fork	meat	sausage	tree
car	fridge	mess	scissors	truck
carpet	fruit	milk	seat	tummy
cat	game	morning	see-saw	wall
chair	garden	mouth	shampoo	washer
cheese	gate	mommy	sheep	watch
chicken	girl	music	shelf	water
children	glass	nail	shirt	wheel
chin	grandma	name	shoe	wind
chocolate	grandpa	nanna	shop	window
circle	grass	nappy/diaper	shower	wood

Pronunciation key to phonetic symbols

Vowels	
/i/	feet
/ɪ/	bit
/ɛ/	get
/æ/	hat
/ɑ/	palm
/ɔ/	jaw
/U/	book
/u/	cool
/ʌ/	but

Diphthongs	
/eɪ/	late
/aɪ/	bite
/aU/	mouse
/oU/	boat
/ɔɪ/	boy
/ɪu/	cute

Consonants	
/p/	pie
/b/	ball
/m/	mess
/w/	water
/f/	fish
/v/	very
/θ/	thin
/ð/	this
/t/	ten
/d/	dog
/n/	no
/s/	soap
/z/	zip
/r/	roof
/l/	lamb
/ʃ/	shoe
/ʒ/	measure
/j/	yes
/k/	key
/g/	girl
/ŋ/	sing
/h/	help

Affricates	
/t ʃ/	cheese
/d ʒ/	jump

Glossary

Adaptive assessment	Assessment procedure in which an examiner compensates for a child's auditory errors by providing: shorter distance, greater voice level, repetition, clarification, context, and/or visible cues; the examiner reports the condition under which a correct response occurred.
Adaptive instruction	Teaching procedure in which instructional methods are selected and modified according to the child's current needs, in order to maximize learning opportunities.
Aided threshold	Weakest sound (e.g., a test tone) a child can detect, when the sound is presented through a loudspeaker, and the child listens through a personal amplification system such as a hearing aid or cochlear implant.
Alveolar	Articulated with the tip of the tongue touching or near the gum ridge behind the upper front teeth (e.g., the consonants /t, d, n, s, z/).
Articulation	Movements and points of contact of the lips, teeth, and tongue during the production of speech.
Assertion	Type of sentence that expresses a request or command, an opinion, a want or need, or a description, commonly called a "statement".
Audiogram	Graph that shows a child's hearing thresholds (decibels relative to normal hearing: "Hearing Level") for test tones of different frequencies (Hertz).
Auditory	Related to the attentive process of listening and/or the perceptual process of hearing.
Auditory-oral	Therapeutic method in which a hearing-impaired child is taught to use available hearing; lipreading is permitted and may even be encouraged.

Auditory (re)habilitation	Process that includes identifying/diagnosing a child's hearing impairment, providing and maintaining hearing aids/cochlear implants, and applying various therapy/teaching methods to help the child attain his/her potential for speech communication.
Auditory-verbal	Therapeutic method in which a hearing-impaired child is taught to use available hearing; lipreading is discouraged to maximize attention to sound and listening.
Bilabial	Articulated mainly by closing or partly closing the lips (e.g., the speech sounds /p, b, m, w/).
Binaural	Related to the perception of sound with both ears.
Choice question	Type of question that limits response alternatives by explicitly naming a small set of items (e.g., "Do you want an apple, orange, or banana?").
Clarification strategy	Remedial action that is applied after a child has misunderstood all or part of a spoken message (e.g., repeat, speak louder/more slowly, simplify).
Clear speech	Production of an utterance with careful articulation, slightly slower than normal rate, and moderate emphasis of key words.
Closed set	Listening task in which a child must choose from a small number of alternatives (e.g., four pictures).
Cochlea	Inner ear structure that contains the sensory mechanism of hearing; the cochlea converts mechanical vibrations from the middle ear into nerve impulses.
Cochlear implant	Small, but complex, hearing device that contains a miniature microphone, digital speech processor, and multiple electrodes surgically implanted in the cochlea; the implant restores sensation and perception of sound to a child with a significant hearing loss.
Communication breakdown	Misunderstanding that has occurred during a conversation, characterized by an inappropriate response, silence, and/or request for clarification.
Communication partner	One of two people participating in a conversational exchange.
Consonant	Speech sound produced by partial or complete closure of the vocal tract.
Context	All circumstances, events, or parts of discourse that precede, follow, or otherwise surround a person's attempt to communicate.
Continuant consonant	Unit of speech in which the sound quality changes little throughout its duration (e.g., nasals, liquids, fricatives).

Decibel	Measure of sound level relative to some reference (e.g., zero decibels Hearing Level = decibels relative to "normal hearing"); commonly abbreviated as dB.
Diagnostic teaching	Activity in which instruction and diagnosis are combined into one process; the use of a child's current performance to plan future learning activities.
Digital signal processing	Method for converting an analog signal, such as an acoustic speech wave into digital (numerical) form, and then modifying the digital signal according to mathematical formulas and rules.
Diphthong	Sequence of two vowels within the same syllable (e.g., eI, aI, ju, oU, aU, oI, as in the words *late, mine, you, soap, cow, toy*).
Effective hearing distance	Range within which a child perceives speech best, and beyond which many sounds are heard with difficulty or not at all.
Fading	Gradual withdrawal of a prompt or cue that was used to help a child learn; transfer of behavior from one controlling stimulus to another.
Formant	Concentration of sound energy in a narrow band of frequencies, related to vocal tract resonance, and typical of vowels and continuant consonants.
Frequency	Number of times an event (e.g., a pressure pulse) repeats within a particular time interval (e.g., a second).
Frequency compression/ transposition	Method for converting speech energy in a higher frequency region to energy in a lower frequency region to make perception easier for a child with a high-frequency hearing loss.
Hearing aid	Small amplification device that contains a miniature microphone, amplifier, earphone, and is powered by a battery; worn on or in the ear; provides audible sound to a child with impaired hearing.
Iambic	Speech pattern in which an unstressed syllable is followed by a stressed syllable (e.g., as in the word *giraffe*).
Intonation	Variation of voice pitch while a person is speaking.
Language	Shared system of symbols that people use to convey ideas, feelings, and concepts.
Lipreading	Method for acquiring speech information by watching the mouth and face of a speaker for visible patterns, articulatory positions/movements, and facial expressions; also referred to as "speechreading".
Manner of articulation	Description of how the breath stream is obstructed to produce a consonant sound (e.g., stop/plosive, nasal, fricative).

Mapping	Adjustments made to the digital signal processor and electrode outputs of a cochlear implant to optimize a child's perception of speech, music, or other sounds.
Medial consonant	Speech sound that occurs between two vowels (e.g., the consonant /m/ in the word *emu*).
Metalinguistic	Conscious awareness of the form and structure of language and how these factors relate to and produce meaning.
Model	To demonstrate a behavior or a sample of spoken language to a child.
Multi-band compression	Method of speech processing in which sound is divided into adjacent frequency bands whose characteristics are processed separately before they are re-combined for presentation to the ears of a hearing-impaired child.
Narrative	Several closely related sentences that are spoken in succession to describe an activity, or tell a story.
Non-verbal cue	Linguistic information conveyed without vocalization or speech (e.g., a nod ("yes"), head shake ("no"), smile, or yawn).
Open set	Listening task in which a child must choose from an unlimited number of alternatives.
Personal listening system	Small, portable electronic device that enables a hearing-impaired child to perceive sound (e.g., hearing aid, cochlear implant).
Phoneme	Smallest audible unit of spoken language that can convey a change in meaning (e.g., as in *bat* vs *mat*).
Phonological system	Child's organization and use of sound for meaningful communication.
Place of articulation	Point of contact (e.g., lips, teeth, palate) between parts of the mouth during production of a consonant sound.
Positive reinforcement	Reward given after a correct response, which increases the probability that the child will repeat this behavior in the future.
Post-dental articulation	Point of contact of the tongue behind the teeth during production of the consonants /t, d, n, l, k, g, ŋ/.
Prosody	Rhythm, stress, and intonation of connected speech.
Redundancy	Condition where a phrase or sentence contains many similar or related words, which results in high predictability (e.g., "The bird flew to its nest.").

Reverberation	Persistence of sound in a room after the original sound has stopped; sound reflects off hard surfaces, producing many echoes.
Role-play	Acting as if you were a character in a situation or story to help a child practice communication skills in a realistic setting.
Semantics	Associations between words and their meanings.
Sensori-neural hearing loss	Hearing impairment in which the site of lesion is the inner ear or auditory nerve, caused by heredity, congenital factors, disease, trauma, or aging.
Soundfield system	Classroom amplification system that uses a wireless microphone, a receiver/amplifier, and loudspeakers to increase a teacher's voice level about 10-15 dB throughout the room.
Spectrum	Distribution of sound energy as a function of frequency.
Speech area	Range of frequencies and intensities typical of ordinary speech at a conversational (one metre) distance, often expressed in dB Hearing Level (HL) and depicted on an audiogram as a distinct region.
Speech feature	Characteristic of a speech sound that distinguishes it from other, similar speech sounds such as voicing, nasality, frication, etc.
Speech processor	Miniature computer within a hearing aid or cochlear implant designed to modify speech for delivery to the ear of a hearing-impaired child.
Speech-to-noise ratio	Difference (in decibels) between the sound level of a person's speech and that of background noise; often abbreviated as S/N or SNR.
Spoken language	Acoustic method of communication commonly referred to as "speech".
Spondee	Word consisting of two stressed syllables (e.g., as in the word *toothbrush*).
Stop consonant	Unit of speech whose sound quality changes throughout its duration, produced by a brief closure of the vocal tract (e.g., /p, t, k, b, d, g/).
Supra-segmental	Related to the voice pattern superimposed on a spoken word, phrase, or sentence (e.g., syllable stress, rhythm, or intonation).
Syllable stress	Relative emphasis given to a spoken syllable in loudness, pitch, and/or duration.
Syntax	Rules for word order within a phrase or sentence.

Tactile	Related to sensation through the skin.
Tactile vibrator	Small hand-held device that converts electrical signals (as from speech) into vibratory patterns for presentation to the skin surface.
Threshold	Smallest detectable sensation of sound, often expressed in decibels relative to normal hearing (usually described as "Hearing Level").
Trochaic	Speech pattern in which a stressed syllable is followed by an unstressed syllable (e.g., as in the word *pocket*).
Unaided threshold	Weakest sound (e.g., a test tone) that a child can detect, when the sound is presented through an audiometer and headphones, rather than through a personal listening system such as a hearing aid or cochlear implant.
Velar	Articulated with the back of the tongue touching or near the soft palate (e.g., the consonants /k, g, ŋ/).
Viseme	Smallest visible unit of spoken language that can convey a change in meaning (e.g., as in *map* vs *mat*); a distinctive, visible mouth shape.
Vowel	Speech sound produced with voice, with acoustic characteristics determined by resonances of the vocal tract.
Wh-question	Type of question that limits response alternatives by requesting a specific type of information (e.g., beginning with *who, what, where, when*).
Word association	Process by which a word evokes a strong memory or image of another word (e.g., what word do you think of when you hear the word *sheep*? ... probably one of these words: *lamb, wool,* or *goat*).
Yes/no question	Type of question that limits response alternatives by enquiring whether an implied statement is true or not (e.g., "Did you break the glass?" = "You broke the glass. Is that true?").

References

Abraham, S. (1989). Using a phonological framework to describe speech errors of orally trained, hearing-impaired school-agers. *Journal of Speech and Hearing Disorders, 54*, 600–609.

Alich, G.W. (1967). Language communication by lipreading. In *Proceedings of the International Conference on Oral Education of the Deaf.* Washington, DC: A.G. Bell Association for the Deaf, 465–482.

Allen, M.C., Nikolopoulos, T.P., & O'Donoghue, G.M. (1998). Speech intelligibility in children after cochlear implantation. *Otology & Neurotology, 19*, 742–746.

Allum, J.H.J., Greisiger, R., Straubhaar, S., & Carpenter, M.G. (2000). Auditory perception and speech identification in children with cochlear implants tested with the EARS protocol. *British Journal of Audiology, 34*, 293–303.

Alyeshmerni, M., & Taubr, P. (1975). *Working with aspects of language, (2nd ed.).* New York: Harcourt Brace Jovanovich.

Anderson, I., Baumgartner, W.D., Boheim, K., Nahler, A., Arnoldner, C., & D'Haese, P. (2006). Telephone use: What benefit do cochlear implant users receive? *International Journal of Audiology, 45*, 446–453.

Archbold, S.M., Nikolopoulos, T.P., & Lloyd-Richmond, H. (2009). Long-term use of cochlear implant systems in paediatric recipients and factors contributing to non-use. *Cochlear Implants International, 10*, 25–40.

Argyle, M. (1988). *Bodily communication (2nd ed.).* New York: Methuen.

Armitage, I.M., Burke, J.P., & Buffin, J.T. (1995). Visual impairment in severe and profound sensorineural deafness. *Archives of Disease in Childhood, 73*, 53–56.

Asp, C.W. (1973). The Verbo-Tonal Method as an alternative to present auditory training techniques. In J.W. Wingo & G.F. Holloway (Eds.), *An appraisal of speech pathology and audiology*, Springfield, IL: Thomas.

Auriemmo, J., Kuk, F., Lau, C., Marshall, S., Thiele, N., Pikora, M., Quick, D., & Stenger, P. (2009). Effect of linear frequency transposition on speech recognition and production of school-age children. *Journal of the American Academy of Audiology, 20*, 289–305.

Bankaitis, A.U. (2008). Hearing assistance technology (HAT). In M. Valente, H. Hosford-Dunn & R.J. Roeser (Eds.), *Audiology treatment (2nd ed.).* New York: Thieme, 400–417.

Beattie, R.G. (2006). The oral methods and spoken language acquisition. In P. E. Spencer & M. Marschark (Eds.), *Advances in the development of spoken language by deaf children.* Oxford: Oxford University Press.

Beebe, H.H. (1953). *A guide to help the severely hard of hearing child.* Basel: Karger.

Bekesy, G.V. (1947). A new audiometer. *Acta Otolaryngologica, 35*, 411–422.

Bench, J., Kowal, A., & Bamford, J. (1979). The BKB (Bamford-Kowal-Bench) sentence lists for partially-hearing children. *British Journal of Audiology, 13,* 108–112.

Berger, K.W., & Popelka, G.R. (1971). Extra-facial gestures in relation to speechreading. *Journal of Communication Disorders, 3,* 302–308.

Bergeson, T.R., Pisoni, D.B., & Davis, R.A.O. (2004). A longitudinal study of audiovisual speech perception by children with hearing loss who have cochlear implants. *Volta Review, 103 (4), monograph,* 347–370.

Berlin, C.I. (2007). A listener's guide to the hearing loss simulation CD. In S. Schwartz (Ed.), *Choices in deafness: A parent's guide to communication options (3rd ed.).* Bethesda, MD: Woodbine House.

Berlin, C.I., Keats, B.J.B., Hood, L.J., Gregory, P., & Rance, G. (2007). Auditory neuropathy/dys-synchrony (AN/AD). In S. Schwartz (Ed.), *Choices in deafness: A parent's guide to communication options (3rd ed.).* Bethesda, MD: Woodbine House, 49–62.

Bernstein, L.E., Goldstein, M.H., & Mahshie, J.J. (1988). Speech training aids for hearing-impaired individuals: I. Overview and aims. *Journal of Rehabilitation Research and Development, 25,* 53–62.

Binnie, C.A. (1976). Relevant aural rehabilitation. In J. Northern (Ed.), *Hearing disorders.* Boston, MA: Little Brown, 213–227.

Blamey, P., & Sarant, J. (2002). Speech perception and language criteria for pediatric cochlear implant candidature. *Audiology and Neuro-Otology, 7,* 114–121.

Blamey, P.J., Sarant, J.Z., Paatsch, L.E., Barry, J.G., Bow, C.P., Wales, R.J., Wright, M., Psarros, C., Rattigan, K., & Tooher, R. (2001). Relationships among speech perception, production, language, hearing loss, and age in children with impaired hearing. *Journal of Speech-Language Hearing Research, 44,* 264–285.

Bode, D.L., & Carhart, R. (1974). Stability and accuracy of adaptive tests of speech discrimination. *Journal of the Acoustical Society of America, 56,* 963–970.

Bones, C., & Diggory, S. (1999). An evaluation of one cochlear implant user's speech perception: With and without an FM system and lip-pattern in controlled background noise levels. *Deafness and Education International, 1,* 83–95.

Boothroyd, A. (1968). Developments in speech audiometry. *Sound, 2,* 3–10.

Boothroyd, A. (1971). Acoustics of speech. In L.E. Connor (Ed.), *Speech for the deaf child: Knowledge and use.* Washington, DC: A.G. Bell Association for the Deaf, 3–44. Key to phonetic symbols.

Boothroyd, A. (1984). Auditory perception of speech contrasts by subjects with sensorineural hearing loss. *Journal of Speech and Hearing Research, 27,* 134–144.

Boothroyd, A. (1991). Assessment of speech perception capacity in profoundly deaf children. *American Journal of Otology, 12,* S67–S72.

Boothroyd, A., & Boothroyd-Turner, D. (2002). Post-implant audition and educational attainment in children with prelingually-acquired profound deafness. *Annals of Otology, Rhinology, and Laryngology, 111 (Suppl. 189),* 79–84.

Boothroyd, A., & Eran, O. (1994). Auditory speech perception capacity of child implant users expressed as equivalent hearing loss. *Volta Review, 96 (5, monograph),* 151–167.

Boothroyd, A., Geers, A.E., & Moog, J.S. (1991). Practical implications of cochlear implants in children. *Ear and Hearing, 12,* 81S–89S.

Boothroyd, A., Springer, N., Smith, L., & Schulman, J. (1988). Amplitude compression and profound hearing loss. *Journal of Speech and Hearing Research, 31,* 362–376.

Bradlow, A.R., Kraus, N., & Hayes, E. (2003). Speaking clearly for children with learning disabilities: Sentence perception in noise. *Journal of Speech, Language, and Hearing Research, 46,* 80–97.

REFERENCES

Butt, D.S., & Chreist, F.M. (1968). A speechreading test for young children. *Volta Review, 70,* 225–239.

Caissie, R., Campbell, M.M., Frenette, W.L., Scott, L., Howell, I., & Roy, A. (2005). Clear speech for adults with a hearing loss: Does intervention with communication partners make a difference? *Journal of the American Academy of Audiology, 16,* 157–171.

Caissie, R., & Wilson, E. (1995). Communication breakdown management during cooperative learning activities by mainstreamed students with hearing losses. *Volta Review, 97,* 105–121.

Calderon, R. (2000). Parental involvement in deaf children's education programs as a predictor of child's language, early reading, and social-emotional development. *Journal of Deaf Studies and Deaf Education, 5(2),* 140–155.

Caleffe-Schenck, N., & Baker, D. (2008). *Speech sounds: A guide for parents and professionals.* Centennial, CO: Cochlear Americas.

Calmels, M.N., Saliba, I., Wanna, G., Cochard, N., Fillaux, J., Deguine, O., & Fraysse, B. (2004). Speech perception and speech intelligibility in children after cochlear implantation. *International Journal of Pediatric Otorhinolaryngology, 68,* 347–351.

Calvert, D.R. (1962). Speech sound duration and the surd-sonant error. *Volta Review, 64,* 401–403.

Calvert, D.R., & Silverman, S.R. (1975). *Speech and deafness: A text for learning and teaching.* Washington, DC: A.G. Bell Association.

Carney, A.E. (1986). Understanding speech intelligibility in the hearing impaired. *Topics in Language Disorders, 16,* 47–59.

Castle, D.L. (1978). Telephone communication for the hearing impaired: Methods and equipment. *Journal of the Academy of Rehabilitative Audiology, 11,* 91–104.

Castle, D.L. (1988). *Telephone strategies: A technical and practical guide for hard-of-hearing people.* Bethesda, MD: Self Help for Hard of Hearing People.

Chermak, G.D. (1981). *Handbook of audiological rehabilitation.* Springfield, IL: Thomas.

Chermak, G.D., & Musiek, F.E. (2002). Auditory training: Principles and approaches for remediating and managing auditory processing disorders. *Seminars in Hearing, 23,* 297–308.

Chute, P.M., & Nevins, M.E. (2002). *The parents' guide to cochlear implants.* Washington, DC: Gallaudet University Press.

Clark, H.H., & Clark, E.V. (1977). *Psychology and language.* New York: Harcourt Brace Jovanovich.

Clezy, G. (1984). An early auditory-oral intervention program. In D. Ling (Ed.), *Early intervention for hearing-impaired children: Oral options.* San Diego, CA: College-Hill Press, 65–117.

Clouser, R.A. (1976). The effect of vowel-consonant ratio and sentence length on lipreading ability. *American Annals of the Deaf, 121,* 513–518.

Cohen, D. (2006). *The development of play (3rd ed.).* London: Routledge.

Cole, E., & Flexer, C. (2011). *Children with hearing loss: Developing listening and talking, birth to six (2nd ed.).* San Diego: Plural Publishing.

Compton, C.L. (2000). Assistive technology for the enhancement of receptive communication. In J.G. Alpiner & P.A. McCarthy (Eds.), *Rehabilitative audiology: Children and adults (3rd ed.).* Philadelphia: Lippincott, 501–555.

Crandell, C.C., & Smaldino, J. (2002). Room acoustics and auditory rehabilitation technology. In J. Katz (Ed.), *Handbook of clinical audiology (5th ed.).* London: Lippincott, Williams & Wilkins.

Crandell, C.C., Smaldino, J.J., & Flexer, C., (Eds.) (2005). *Sound field amplification: Applications to speech perception and classroom acoustics (2nd ed.)*. Clifton Park, NY: Thomson Delmar Learning.

Cray, J.W., Allen, R.L., Stuart, A., Hudson, S., Layman, E., & Givens, G.D. (2004). An investigation of telephone use among cochlear implant recipients. *American Journal of Audiology, 13*, 200–212.

Dagenais, P.A., Critz-Crosby, P., Fletcher, S.G., & McCutcheon, M.J. (1994). Comparing abilities of children with profound hearing impairment to learn consonants using electropalatography or traditional aural-oral techniques. *Journal of Speech and Hearing Research, 37*, 687–699.

Dawson, P.W., Nott, P.E., Clark, G.M., & Cowan, R.S.C. (1998). A modification of play audiometry to assess speech discrimination ability in severe-profoundly deaf 2- to 4-year-old children. *Ear and Hearing, 19*, 371–384.

De Filippo, C.L. (1982). Memory for articulated sequences and lipreading performance of hearing-impaired observers. *Volta Review, 84*, 134–145.

De Filippo, C.L. (1988). Tracking for speechreading training. In C.L. De Filippo & D.G. Sims (Eds.), New reflections on speechreading. *Volta Review, 90*, 215–239.

De Filippo, C.L., & Scott, B.L. (1978). A method for training and evaluating the reception of ongoing speech. *Journal of the Acoustical Society of America, 63*, 1186–1192.

Demorest, M.E. (1986). Problem-solving: Stages, strategies, and stumbling blocks. *Journal of the Academy of Rehabilitative Audiology, 19*, 13–26.

DesJardin, J.L., & Eisenberg, L.S. (2007). Maternal contributions: Supporting language development in young children with cochlear implants. *Ear and Hearing, 28*, 456–469.

Dillon, H. (2001). *Hearing aids*. New York: Thieme.

Dornan, D., Hickson, L., Murdoch, B., Houston, T., & Constantinescu, G. (2010). Is auditory-verbal therapy effective for children with hearing loss? *Volta Review, 110*, 361–387.

Duncan, S. (1972). Some signals and rules for taking speaking turns in conversations. *Journal of Personality and Social Psychology, 23*, 283–292.

Easterbrooks, S.R., & Estes, E.L. (2007). *Helping deaf and hard of hearing students to use spoken language*. Thousand Oaks, CA: Corwin Press.

Eisenberg, L. (2007). Current state of knowledge: Speech recognition and production in children with hearing impairment. *Ear and Hearing, 28*, 766–772.

Eisenberg, L.S., Martinez, A.S., Holowecky, S.R., & Pogorelsky, S. (2002). Recognition of lexically controlled words and sentences by children with normal hearing and children with cochlear implants. *Ear and Hearing, 23*, 450–462.

Elliott, L.L., & Katz, D.R. (1980). Northwestern University Children's Perception of Speech Test (NUCHIPS). St. Louis, MO: Auditec.

Entwisle, D.R. (1966). *Word associations of young children*. Baltimore, MD: Johns Hopkins Press.

Erber, N.P. (1971). Effects of distance on the visual reception of speech. *Journal of Speech and Hearing Research, 14*, 848–857.

Erber, N.P. (1972a). Auditory, visual, and auditory-visual recognition of consonants by children with normal and impaired hearing. *Journal of Speech and Hearing Research, 15*, 413–422.

Erber, N.P. (1972b). Speech-envelope cues as an acoustic aid to lipreading for profoundly deaf children. *Journal of the Acoustical Society of America, 51*, 1224–1227.

Erber, N.P. (1974a). Effects of angle, distance, and illumination on visual reception of speech by profoundly deaf children. *Journal of Speech and Hearing Research, 17*, 99–112.

Erber, N.P. (1974b). Pure-tone thresholds and word-recognition abilities of hearing-impaired children. *Journal of Speech and Hearing Research, 17*, 194–202.

REFERENCES

Erber, N.P. (1975). Auditory-visual perception of speech. *Journal of Speech and Hearing Disorders, 40,* 481–492.

Erber, N.P. (1976). The use of audio tape-cards in auditory training for hearing-impaired children. *Volta Review, 78,* 209–221.

Erber, N.P. (1977). Developing materials for lipreading evaluation and instruction. *Volta Review, 79,* 35–42.

Erber, N.P. (1978). Vibratory perception by deaf children. *International Journal of Rehabilitation Research, 1,* 27–37.

Erber, N.P. (1979a). Auditory-visual perception of speech with reduced optical clarity. *Journal of Speech and Hearing Research, 22,* 212–223.

Erber, N.P. (1979b). Speech perception by profoundly hearing-impaired children. *Journal of Speech and Hearing Disorders, 44,* 255–270.

Erber, N.P. (1980a). Auditory evaluation and training of hearing-impaired children. *Journal of the National Student Speech and Hearing Association, 8,* 6–18.

Erber, N.P. (1980b). Speech correction through the use of acoustic models. In J.D. Subtelny (Ed.), *Speech assessment and speech improvement for the hearing-impaired.* Washington, DC: A.G. Bell Association for the Deaf, 222–241.

Erber, N.P. (1982). *Auditory training.* Washington, DC: A.G. Bell Association for the Deaf.

Erber, N.P. (1984). *QUEST?AR. (Questions for Aural Rehabilitation).* Abbotsford, Vic. (Australia): Clavis.

Erber, N.P. (1985). *Telephone communication and hearing impairment.* San Diego, CA: College-Hill Press.

Erber, N.P. (1988). *Communication therapy for hearing-impaired adults.* Abbotsford, Vic. (Australia): Clavis.

Erber, N.P. (1992a). Adaptive assessment of adult sentence perception. *Ear and Hearing, 13,* 58–60.

Erber, N.P. (1992b). Effects of a question-answer format on visual perception of sentences. *Journal of the Academy of Rehabilitative Audiology, 25,* 113–122.

Erber, N.P. (1993). *Communication and adult hearing loss.* Abbotsford, Vic. (Australia): Clavis.

Erber, N.P. (1995). Applications of hearing-loss simulation in education of student clinicians. *Journal of the Academy of Rehabilitative Audiology, 28,* 37–50.

Erber, N.P. (1996). *Communication therapy for adults with sensory loss (2nd ed.).* Clifton Hill, Vic. (Australia): Clavis.

Erber, N.P. (1998). DYALOG: A computer-based measure of conversational performance. *Journal of the Academy of Rehabilitative Audiology, 31,* 69–76.

Erber, N.P. (2002). *Hearing, vision, communication, and older people.* Clifton Hill, Vic. (Australia): Clavis.

Erber, N.P. (2008). *Hearing-loss simulation: Education, training, research.* Clifton Hill, Vic. (Australia): Helosonics.

Erber, N.P., & Alencewicz, C.M. (1976). Audiologic evaluation of deaf children. *Journal of Speech and Hearing Disorders, 41,* 256–267.

Erber, N.P., & Greer, C.W. (1973). Communication strategies used by teachers at an oral school for the deaf. *Volta Review, 75,* 480–485.

Erber, N.P., & Hirsh, I.J. (1978). Auditory training. In H. Davis & S.R. Silverman (Eds.), *Hearing and Deafness (4th ed.).* New York, NY: Holt, Rinehart, and Winston, 358–374.

Erber, N.P., & Lamb, N.L. (1995). Situ-Action: Teaching students to identify client needs with conversational scenarios. *Journal of the Academy of Rehabilitative Audiology, 28,* 51–59.

Erber, N.P., & Lind, C. (1994). Communication therapy: Theory and practice. In J-P Gagné & N. Tye-Murray (Eds.), Research in audiological rehabilitation, *Journal of the Academy of Rehabilitative Audiology, 27 (Monog. Suppl.)*, 267–287.

Erber, N.P., & McMahon, D.A. (1976). Effects of sentence context on recognition of words through lipreading by deaf children. *Journal of Speech and Hearing Research, 19,* 112–119.

Erber, N.P., & Witt, L. (1977). Effects of stimulus intensity on speech perception by deaf children. *Journal of Speech and Hearing Disorders, 42,* 271–278.

Erber, N.P., & Yelland, J. (1998). CONAN: A system for analysis of temporal factors in conversation. *Journal of the Academy of Rehabilitative Audiology, 31,* 77–86.

Erber, N.P., & Zeiser, M.L. (1974). Classroom observation under conditions of simulated profound deafness. *Volta Review, 76,* 352–360.

Ertmer, D.J., Young, N.M., & Nathani, S. (2007). Profiles of vocal development in young cochlear implant recipients. *Journal of Speech, Language, and Hearing Research, 50,* 393–407.

Estabrooks, W. (1994). *Auditory-verbal therapy for parents and professionals.* Washington, DC: A.G. Bell Association.

Estabrooks, W. (Ed.) (2006). *Auditory-verbal therapy and practice.* Washington, DC: A.G. Bell Association.

Estabrooks, W., & Birkenshaw-Fleming, L. (Eds.) (2003). *Songs for listening! Songs for life!* Washington, DC: A.G. Bell Association.

Ewing, I.R., & Ewing, A.W.G. (1961). *New opportunities for deaf children.* London: University of London Press.

Finitzo-Hieber, T., & Tillman, T.W. (1978). Room acoustics effects on monosyllabic word discrimination ability for normal and hearing-impaired children. *Journal of Speech and Hearing Research, 21,* 440–458.

Fletcher, H. (1929). *Speech and hearing.* New York: Van Nostrand.

Flexer, C. (1999). *Facilitating hearing and listening in young children (2nd ed.).* San Diego, CA: Singular Press.

Flipsen, P., & Colvard, L.G. (2006). Intelligibility of conversational speech produced by children with cochlear implants. *Journal of Communication Disorders, 39,* 93–108.

Flynn, M.C., & Dowell, R.C. (1999). Speech perception in a communicative context: An investigation using question/answer pairs. *Journal of Speech, Language, and Hearing Research, 42,* 540–552.

Franz, D.C., Caleffe-Schenck, N., & Kirk, K.I. (2004). A tool for assessing functional use of audition in children: Results in children with the MED-EL COMBI 40+ cochlear implant system. *Volta Review, 104,* 175–196.

Gagné, J-P., & Erber, N.P. (1987). Simulation of sensorineural hearing impairment. *Ear and Hearing, 8,* 232–243.

Gagné, J-P, Masterson, V., Munhall, K.G., Bilida, N., & Querengesser, C. (1994). Across-talker variability in auditory, visual, and audiovisual speech intelligibility for conversational and clear speech. *Journal of the Academy of Rehabilitative Audiology, 27,* 135–158.

Galvin, K.L., Ginis, J., Cowan, R.S.C., Blamey, P.J., & Clark, G.M. (2001). A comparison of a new prototype Tickle Talker with the Tactaid 7. *Australian and New Zealand Journal of Audiology, 23,* 18–36.

Garstecki, D.C., & O'Neill, J.J. (1980). Situational cue and strategy influence on speechreading. *Scandinavian Audiology, 9,* 147–151.

Gault, R.H. (1927), "Hearing" through the sense organs of touch and vibration. *Journal of the Franklin Institute, 204,* 329–358.

Gault, R.H. (1930). A partial analysis of the effects of tactual-visual stimulation by spoken language. *Journal of the Franklin Institute, 209,* 437–458.

REFERENCES

Gault, R.H. (1936). Recent developments in vibro-tactile research. *Journal of the Franklin Institute, 221,* 703–719.

Geers, A.E. (2006). Factors influencing spoken language outcomes in children following early cochlear implantation. *Advances in Otorhinolaryngology, 64,* 50–65.

Geers, A., Brenner, C., & Davidson, L. (2003a). Factors associated with development of speech perception skills in children implanted by age 5. *Ear and Hearing, 24 (Suppl),* 24S–35S.

Geers, A.E., & Hayes, H. (2011). Reading, writing, and phonological processing skills of adolescents with 10 or more years of cochlear implant experience. *Ear and Hearing, 32 (Suppl),* 49S–59S.

Geers, A.E., Nicholas, J.G., & Sedey, A.L. (2003b). Language skills of children with early cochlear implantation. *Ear and Hearing, 24 (Suppl),* 46S–58S.

Geers, A.E., & Sedey, A.L (2011). Language and verbal reasoning skills in adolescents with 10 or more years of cochlear implant experience. *Ear and Hearing, 32 (Suppl),* 39S–48S.

Geers, A.E., Strube, M.J., Tobey, E.A., Pisoni, D.B., & Moog, J.S. (2011). Epilogue: Factors contributing to long-term outcomes of cochlear implantation in early childhood. *Ear and Hearing, 32 (Suppl),* 84S–92S.

Glista, D., Scollie, S., Bagatto, M., Seewald, R., Parsa, V., & Johnson, A. (2009). Evaluation of nonlinear frequency compression: Clinical outcomes. *International Journal of Audiology, 48,* 632–644.

Gnosspelius, J., & Spens, K-E (1992). A computer-based speech tracking procedure. STL-QPSR (KTH, Stockholm), *1,* 131–137.

Goldberg, D.M. (1988). Auditory tracking by hearing-impaired preschoolers: Two case studies. *Journal of the Academy of Rehabilitative Audiology, 21,* 43–48.

Goldstein, M.A. (1939). *The acoustic method.* St Louis, MO: Laryngoscope Press.

Golf, H.R. (1970). Speech through auditory training. In *Report of the Proceedings of the 44th Meeting of the Convention of American Instructors of the Deaf.* Washington, DC: U.S. Government Printing Office.

Grant, K.W., & Seitz, P-F. (2000). The use of visible speech cues for improving auditory detection of spoken sentences. *Journal of the Acoustical Society of America, 108,* 1197–1208.

Greenspan, S., Burka, A., Zlotow, S., & Barenboim, C. (1975). A manual of referential communication games. *Academic Therapy, 11,* 97–106.

Grice, H.P. (1975). Logic and conversation. In P. Cole & J.L. Morgan (Eds.), *Syntax and semantics 3: Speech acts.* New York, NY: Academic Press, 41–58.

Griffiths, C. (1967). *Conquering childhood deafness.* New York: Exposition Press.

Groht, M.A. (1958). *Natural language for deaf children.* Washington, DC: A.G. Bell Association for the Deaf.

Gstoettner, W.K., Hamzavi, J., Egelierier, B., & Baumgartner, W.D. (2000). Speech perception performance in prelingually deaf children with cochlear implants. *Acta Oto-Laryngologica, 120,* 209–213.

Guberina, P. (1964). Verbotonal method and its application to the rehabilitation of the deaf. *Proceedings of the International Congress on Education of the Deaf.* Washington, DC: U.S. Government Printing Office.

Hack, Z.C., & Erber, N.P. (1982). Auditory, visual, and auditory-visual perception of vowels by hearing-impaired children. *Journal of Speech and Hearing Research, 25,* 100–107.

Harkins, J.E., & Bakke, M. (2003). Technologies for communication: Status and trends. In M. Marschark & P.E. Spencer (Eds.), *Oxford handbook of deaf studies, language, and education.* New York, NY: Oxford University Press, 406–409.

Harrigan, S., & Nikolopoulos, T.P. (2002). Parent interaction course in order to increase communication skills between parents and children following pediatric cochlear implantation. *International Journal of Pediatric Otorhinolaryngology, 66(2)*, 161–166.

Haskins, H. (1949). A phonetically balanced test of speech discrimination for children. Masters thesis. Evanston, IL: Northwestern University.

Hedley-Williams, A.J., Sladen, D.P., & Tharpe, A.M. (2003). Programming, care, and troubleshooting of cochlear implants for children. *Topics in Language* Disorders, *23*, 46–56.

Hnath-Chisholm, T.E., Laipply, E., & Boothroyd, A. (1998). Age-related changes on a children's test of sensory-level speech perception capacity. *Journal of Speech, Language, and Hearing Research, 41*, 94–106.

Hopper, R. (1992). *Telephone conversation.* Bloomington, IN: Indiana University Press.

Howard-Jones, P.A., Whybrow, J.J., & Summers, I.R. (2001). An evaluation of an electronic simulation of hearing impairment in the training of mainstream teachers. *European Journal of Special Needs Education, 16*, 277–287.

Hudgins, C.V. (1948). A rationale for acoustic training. *Volta Review, 50*, 484–490.

Hudgins, C.V. (1954). Auditory training: Its possibilities and limitations. *Volta Review, 56*, 339–349.

Hudgins, C.V., Hawkins, J.E., Karlin, J.E., & Stevens, S.S. (1947). The development of recorded auditory tests for measuring hearing loss for speech. *Laryngoscope, 47*, 57–89.

Hudgins, C.V., & Numbers, F.C. (1942). An investigation of intelligibility of the speech of the deaf. *Genetic Psychology Monographs, 25*, 289–392.

Ibertsson, T., Hansson, K., Asker-Arnason, L., & Sahlen, B. (2009). Speech recognition, working memory, and conversation in children with cochlear implants. *Deafness and Education International. 11*, 132–151.

Jeffers, J., & Barley, M. (1971). *Speechreading (Lipreading).* Springfield, IL: Thomas.

Jennings, M.B. (1995). Service delivery models for older adults with hearing impairments: Individual sessions. In P.B. Kricos & S.A. Lesner (Eds.), *Hearing care for the older adult.* Boston: Butterworth-Heinemann, 227–265.

Johansson, B. (1966). The use of the transposer for the management of the deaf child. *International Audiology, 5*, 362–372.

Kalikow, D.N., Stevens, K.N., & Elliott, L.L. (1977). Development of a test of speech intelligibility in noise using sentence materials of controlled word predictability. *Journal of the Acoustical Society of America, 61*, 1337–1351.

Kaplan, H.K., Bally, S.J., & Garretson, C. (1987). *Speechreading: A way to improve understanding (2nd ed.).* Washington, DC: Gallaudet University Press.

Karp, A. (1988). Reduced vision and speechreading. In C.L. De Filippo & D.G. Sims (Eds.), New Reflections on Speechreading. *Volta Review, 90 (Suppl.)*, 61–74.

Kent, R.D. (Ed.) (2004). *The MIT encyclopedia of communication disorders.* Cambridge, MA: MIT Press.

Kenworthy, O.T. (1986). Caregiver–child interaction and language acquisition of hearing-impaired children. *Topics in Language Disorders, 6*, 1–11.

Kepler, L.J, Terry, M., & Sweetman, R.H. (1992). Telephone usage in the hearing-impaired population. *Ear & Hearing, 13*, 311–330.

Kirk, K.I., Pisoni, D.B., & Osberger, M.J. (1995). Lexical effects on spoken word recognition by pediatric cochlear implant users. *Ear and Hearing, 16*, 470–481.

Klieve, S., & Jeanes, R.C. (2001). Perception of prosodic features by children with cochlear implants: Is it sufficient for perceiving meaning differences in language? *Deafness and Education International, 3*, 15–37.

REFERENCES

Kricos, P.B., & Lesner, S.A. (1982). Differences in visual intelligibility across talkers. *Volta Review, 84,* 219–225.

Kuk, F., Keenen, D., Auriemmo, J., Korhonen, P., Peeters, H., Lau, C., & Crose, B. (2010). Interpreting the efficacy of frequency-lowering algorithms. *Hearing Journal, 63,* 30, 32, 34, 36–38, 40.

Lachs, L., Pisoni, D.B., & Kirk, K.I. (2001). Use of audiovisual information in speech perception by prelingually deaf children with cochlear implants: A first report. *Ear and Hearing, 22,* 236–251.

Lane, H.L., & Tranel, B. (1971). The Lombard sign and the role of hearing in speech. *Journal of Speech and Hearing Research, 14,* 677–709.

Levin, S., & Erber, N.P. (1976). A vision screening program for deaf children. *Volta Review, 78,* 90–99.

Levinson, S.C. (1983). *Pragmatics.* Cambridge: Cambridge University Press.

Levitt, H. (1971). Speech production and the deaf child. In L.E. Connor (Ed.), *Speech for the deaf child: Knowledge and use.* Washington, DC: A. G. Bell Association, 59–83.

Levitt, H., McGarr, N.S., & Geffner, D. (Eds.) (1987). Development of language and communication skills of hearing-impaired children. *ASHA Monographs, 26.*

Ling, D. (1964). Implications of hearing aid amplification below 300 cps. *Volta Review, 66,* 723–729.

Ling, D. (1976). *Speech and the hearing-impaired child: Theory and practice.* Washington, DC: A.G. Bell Association.

Ling, D. (1989). *Foundations of spoken language for hearing-impaired children.* Washington, DC: A.G. Bell Association.

Ling, D. (2003). The six-sound test. In W. Estabrooks & L. Birkenshaw-Fleming (Eds.), *Songs for listening! Songs for life!* Washington, DC: A.G. Bell Association for the Deaf, 227–229.

Ling, D., & Ling, A.H. (1978). *Aural habilitation: The foundations of verbal learning in hearing-impaired children.* Washington, DC: A.G. Bell Association for the Deaf.

Lloyd, J. (1999). Hearing-impaired children's strategies for managing communication breakdowns. *Deafness and Education International, 1,* 188–199.

Lloyd, J., Lieven, E., & Arnold, P. (2005). The oral referential communication skills of hearing-impaired children. *Deafness and Education International, 7,* 22–42.

Lloyd, P. (1991). Strategies used to communicate route directions by telephone: A comparison of the performance of 7-year-olds, 10-year-olds, and adults. *Journal of Child Language, 18,* 171–189.

Lloyd, P. (1992). The role of clarification requests in children's communication of route directions by telephone. *Discourse Processes, 15,* 357–374.

Locke, J.L. (1993). *The child's path to spoken language.* Cambridge, MA: Harvard University Press.

Lubinsky, J. (1986). Choosing aural rehabilitation directions: Suggestions from a model of information processing. *Journal of the Academy of Rehabilitative Audiology, 19,* 27–41.

Ludvigsen, C. (1974). Construction and evaluation of an audio-visual test (The Helen Test). *Scandinavian Audiology, 3 (Suppl. 4),* 67–75.

Luterman, D. (1984). *Counselling the communicatively disordered and their families.* Boston, MA: Little Brown.

Maassen, B., & Povel, D.J. (1985). The effect of segmental and suprasegmental corrections on the intelligibility of deaf speech. *Journal of the Acoustical Society of America, 78,* 877–886.

MacIver-Lux, K. (2009). Intervention for children with cochlear implants: Maximizing auditory benefits of bilateral hearing. *Perspectives on Hearing and Hearing Disorders in Childhood, 19,* 85–97.

Mackie, K., & Dermody, P. (1986). Use of a monosyllabic adapative speech test (MAST) with young children. *Journal of Speech and Hearing Research, 29*, 275–281.

Madell, J.R. (1992). FM systems as primary amplification for children with profound hearing loss. *Ear and Hearing, 13*, 102–107.

Madell, J.R. (1996). Speech audiometry for children. Chapter in Gerber, S.E. (Ed.), *Handbook of pediatric audiology*. Washington, DC: Gallaudet University Press.

Maltby, M. (2000). A new speech perception test for profoundly deaf children. *Deafness and Education International, 2*, 86–100.

Markides, A. (1983). *The speech of hearing-impaired children*. Manchester, UK: Manchester University Press.

Marshall, P.J., & Fox, N.A. (Eds.) (2006). *The development of social engagement: Neurobiological perspectives*. New York: Oxford University Press.

McCall, R. (1991). *Hearing loss? A guide to self-help*. London: Robert Hale.

McGarr, N.S. (1983). The intelligibility of deaf speech to experienced and inexperienced listeners. *Journal of Speech and Hearing Research, 26*, 451–458.

McLeod, R., & Guenther, M. (1977). Use of an ordinary telephone by an oral deaf person: A case history. *Volta Review, 79*, 435–442.

Merklein, R.A. (1981). A short speech perception test for severely and profoundly deaf children. *Volta Review, 83*, 36–45.

Meyer, T.A., Svirsky, M.A., Kirk, K.I., & Miyamoto, R.T. (1998). Improvements in speech perception by children with profound prelingual hearing loss. *Journal of Speech, Language, and Hearing Research, 41*, 846–858.

Miller, G.A., Heise, G., & Lichten, W. (1951). The intelligibility of speech as a function of the context of the test materials. *Journal of Experimental Psychology, 41*, 329–335.

Miyamoto, R.T., Kirk, K.I., Robbins, A.M., Todd, S., & Riley, A. (1996). Speech perception and speech production skills of children with multichannel cochlear implants. *Acta Otolaryngologica, 116*, 240–243.

Monsen, R. (1978). Toward measuring how well hearing-impaired children speak. *Journal of Speech and Hearing Research, 21*, 197–219.

Monsen, R.B. (1983a) The oral speech intelligibility of hearing-impaired talkers. *Journal of Speech and Hearing Disorders, 48*, 286–296.

Monsen, R.B. (1983b). General effects of deafness on phonation and articulation. In I. Hochberg, H. Levitt & M.J. Osberger (Eds.), *Speech of the hearing impaired: Research, training, and personnel preparation*. Baltimore, MD: University Park Press, 23–34.

Monsen, R.B., & Shaughnessy, D.H. (1978). Improvement in vowel articulation of deaf children. *Journal of Communication Disorders, 11*, 417–424.

Montgomery, A.A., & Houston, K.T. (2000). The hearing-impaired adult: Management of communication deficits and tinnitus. In J.G. Alpiner & P.A. McCarthy (Eds.), *Rehabilitative audiology: Children and adults (3rd ed.)*. Philadelphia, PA: Lippincott Williams & Wilkins, 377–401.

Moog, J.S. (2002). Changing expectations for children with cochlear implants. *Annals of Otology, Rhinology, and Laryngology, 111, (Suppl. 189)*, 138–142.

Moog, J.S., Biedenstein, J., Davidson, L., & Brenner, C. (1994). Instruction for developing speech perception skills. In A.E. Geers & J.S. Moog (Eds.), Effectiveness of cochlear implants and tactile aids for deaf children: The Sensory Aids Study at Central Institute for the Deaf, *Volta Review, 96, 5 (monograph)*, 61–73.

Moog, J.S., & Geers, A.E. (1985). *Grammatical analysis of elicited language: Simple sentence level (2nd ed.)*. St. Louis, MO: Central Institute for the Deaf.

REFERENCES

Moog, J.S., & Geers, A.E. (1990). *Early speech perception test*. St. Louis, MO: Central Institute for the Deaf.

Morkovin, B.V. (1947). Rehabilitation of the aurally handicapped through the study of speechreading in life situations. *Journal of Speech and Hearing Disorders, 12*, 363–368.

Most, T., & Peled, M. (2007). Perception of suprasegmental features of speech by children with cochlear implants and children with hearing aids. *Journal of Deaf Studies and Deaf Education, 12*, 350–361.

Most, T., & Shurgi, M. (1993). The effect of listeners' experience on the evaluation of intonation contours produced by hearing-impaired children. *Ear and Hearing, 14*, 112–117.

Myllyniemi, R. (1986). Conversation as a system of social interaction. *Language and Communication, 6*, 147–169.

Nejime, Y., & Moore, B.C.J. (1997). Simulation of the effect of threshold elevation and loudness recruitment combined with reduced frequency selectivity on the intelligibility of speech in noise. *Journal of the Acoustical Society of America, 102*, 603–615.

Nelson, P.B., & Soli, S. (2000). Acoustical barriers to learning: Children at risk in every classroom. *Language, Speech, and Hearing Services in Schools, 31*, 356–361.

Nevins, M.E., & Chute, P.M. (1996). *Children with cochlear implants in educational settings*. San Diego, CA: Singular.

Nicholas, J.G., & Geers, A.E. (2006). Effects of early auditory experience on the spoken language of deaf children at three years of age. *Ear and Hearing, 27*, 286–298.

Nickerson, R.S. (1975). Characteristics of the speech of deaf persons. *Volta Review, 77*, 342–362.

Nikolopoulos, T.P., Wells, P., & Archbold, S.M. (2000). Using Listening Progress Profile (LiP) to assess early functional auditory performance in young implanted children. *Deafness and Education International, 2*, 142–151.

Nittrouer, S., & Boothroyd, A. (1990). Context effects in phoneme and word recognition by young children and older adults. *Journal of the Acoustical Society of America, 87*, 2705–2715.

Northern, J.L., & Downs, M.P. (2002). *Hearing in children (5th ed.)*. Baltimore, MD: Lippincott Williams & Wilkins.

Ochs, M.T., Humes, L.E., Ohde, R.N., & Grantham, D.W. (1989). Frequency discrimination ability and stop consonant identification in normally-hearing and hearing-impaired subjects. *Journal of Speech and Hearing Research, 32*, 133–142.

O'Donoghue, G.M., Nikolopoulos, T.P., Archbold, S.M., & Tait, M. (1998). Speech perception in children after cochlear implantation. *American Journal of Otology, 19*, 762–767.

O'Donoghue, G.M., Nikolopoulos, T.P., Archbold, S.M., & Tait, M. (1999). Cochlear implants in young children: The relationship between speech perception and speech intelligibility. *Ear and Hearing, 20*, 419–425.

Oller, D.K. (1980). The emergence of sounds of speech in infancy. In G.H. Yeni-Komshian, J.F. Kavanagh & C.A. Ferguson, (Eds.), *Child phonology, Vol. 1. Production*. New York: Academic Press.

Olsen, W.O., van Tassel, D.J., & Speaks, C.E. (1997). Phoneme and word recognition for words in isolation and in sentences. *Ear and Hearing, 18*, 175–188.

Osberger, M.J., Robbins, A.M., Berry, S.W., Todd, S.L., Hesketh, L.J., & Sedey, A. (1991a). Analysis of the spontaneous speech samples of children with cochlear implants or tactile aids. *American Journal of Otology, 12*, 1515–1545.

Osberger, M.J., Robbins, A.M., Miyamoto, R.T., Berry, S.W., Myers, W.A., Kessler, K.S., & Pope, M.L. (1991b). Speech perception abilities of children with cochlear implants, tactile aids, or hearing aids. *American Journal of Otology, 12 (Suppl.)*, S105–S115.

Owens, E., & Raggio, M. (1987). The UCSF Tracking procedure for evaluation and training of speech reception by hearing- impaired adults. *Journal of Speech and Hearing Disorders, 52*, 120–128.

Owens, E., & Telleen, C.C. (1981) Tracking as an aural rehabilitative process. *Journal of the Academy of Rehabilitative Audiology, 14*, 259–272.

Ozbic, M., & Kogovšek, D. (2010). Vowel formant values in hearing and hearing-impaired children: A discriminant analysis. *Deafness and Education International, 12*, 99–128.

Payton, K.L., Uchanski, R.M., & Braida, L.D. (1994) Intelligibility of conversational and clear speech in noise and reverberation for listeners with normal and impaired hearing. *Journal of the Acoustical Society of America, 95*, 1581–1592.

Pianta, R.C., & Stuhlman, M.W. (2004). Conceptualising risk in relational terms: Associations among the quality of child-adult relationships prior to school entry and children's developmental outcomes in first grade. *Educational and Child Psychology, 21*, 32–45.

Picheny, M.A., Durlach, N.I., & Braida, L.D. (1985). Speaking clearly for the hard of hearing: Intelligibility differences between clear and conversational speech. *Journal of Speech and Hearing Research, 28*, 96–103.

Picheny, M.A., Durlach, N.I., & Braida, L.D. (1986). Speaking clearly for the hard of hearing II: Acoustic characteristics of clear and conversational speech. *Journal of Speech and Hearing Research, 29*, 434–446.

Pickett, J.M. (1999). *The acoustics of speech communication.* Boston: Allyn and Bacon.

Plant, G. (1994). Training in the use of the Tactaid VII: A case study. *KTH STL-QPSR, 35*, 91–102.

Plant, G.L., Macrae, J.H., & Pearce, J.L. (1980). Performance on a lipreading test by native and non-native speakers of English. *Australian Journal of Audiology, 2*, 25–29.

Pollack, D. (1970). *Educational audiology for the limited hearing infant.* Springfield, IL: Thomas.

Pollack, D. (1984). An acoupedic program. In D. Ling (Ed.), *Early intervention for hearing-impaired children: Oral options.* San Diego, CA: College-Hill Press, 181–253.

Pollack, D., Goldberg, D.M., & Caleffe-Schenk, N. (1997). *Educational audiology for the limited hearing infant and preschooler: An auditory-verbal program (3rd ed.).* Springfield, IL: Thomas.

Power, D. (1991). *Understanding hearing loss* (video tape). Brisbane, Qld: Griffith University.

Power, M.R., & Power, D. (2004). Everyone here speaks TXT: Deaf people using SMS in Australia and the rest of the world. *Journal of Deaf Studies and Deaf Education, 9(3)*, 333–343.

Power, M.R., Power, D., & Horstmanshof, L. (2007). Deaf people communicating via SMS, TTY, relay service, fax and computers in Australia. *Journal of Deaf Studies and Deaf Education, 12*, 80–92.

Prince, G. (1982). Narratology: The form and functioning of narrative. *Janua Linguarum. Series Major 108.* Berlin: Mouton.

Rance, G. (Ed.) (2008). *Auditory steady-state response: Generation, recording, and clinical application.* San Diego: Plural.

Rhoades, E.A. (2006). Research outcomes of auditory-verbal intervention: Is the approach justified? *Deafness and Education International, 8*, 125–143.

Rhoades, E.A., & Chisholm, T.H. (2000). Global language progress with an auditory-verbal approach for children who are deaf or hard of hearing. *Volta Review, 102*, 5–24.

Risberg, A., Agelfors, E., & Boberg, G. (1975). Measurements of frequency-discrimination ability of severely and profoundly hearing-impaired children. *KTH Quarterly Progress Report (2-3)*, 40–48.

Romanik, S. (2008). *Auditory skills program for students with hearing impairment.* Sydney, NSW (Australia): Disability Programs – NSW Department of Education and Training.

REFERENCES

Ross, M. (Ed.) (1992). *FM auditory training systems: Characteristics, selection, and use.* Timonium, MD: York Press.

Ross, M., & Lerman, J.W. (1979). A picture identification test for hearing-impaired children. *Journal of Speech and Hearing Research, 13,* 44–53.

Rotteveel, L.J., Snik, A.F., Vermeulen, A.M., Cremers, C.W., & Mylanus, E.A. (2008). Speech perception in congenitally, pre-lingually, and post-lingually deaf children expressed in an equivalent hearing loss value. *Clinical Otolaryngology, 88,* 560–569.

Sacks, H., Schegloff, E.A., & Jefferson, G.A. (1974). A simplest systematics for the organization of turn-taking for conversation. *Language, 50,* 696–735.

Sarant, J.Z., Blamey, P.J., Dowell, R.C., Clark, G.M., & Gibson, W.P.R. (2001). Variation in speech perception scores among children with cochlear implants. *Ear and Hearing, 22,* 18–28.

Schegloff, E.A., & Sacks, H. (1973). Opening up closings. *Semiotica, VIII, 4,* 289–327.

Schery, T.K., & Peters, M.L. (2003). Developing auditory learning in children with cochlear implants. *Topics in Language Disorders, 23,* 4–15.

Schulte, K. (1978). The use of supplementary speech information in verbal communication. *Volta Review, 80,* 12–20.

Schum, D.J. (1996). Intelligibility of clear and conversational speech of young and elderly talkers. *Journal of the American Academy of Audiology, 7,* 212–218.

Schwartz, J.R., & Black, J.W. (1967). Some effects of sentence structure on speechreading. *Central States Speech Journal, 18,* 86–90.

Seewald, R., Moodie, S., Scollie, S., & Bagatto, M. (2005). The DSL method for pediatric hearing instrument fitting: Historical perspective and current issues. *Trends in Amplification, 9,* 145–157.

Shriberg, L.D., & Kwiatkowski, J. (1982). Phonological disorders III: A procedure for assessing severity of involvement. *Journal of Speech and Hearing Disorders, 47,* 256–270.

Simmons, A.A. (1968). Content subjects through language. In H.G. Kopp (Ed.), *Curriculum: Cognition and content.* Washington, DC: A.G. Bell Association for the Deaf., 121–126.

Simmons, A.A. (1971). Language and hearing. In L.E. Connor (Ed.), *Speech for the deaf child: Knowledge and use.* Washington, DC: A.G. Bell Association for the Deaf, 280–292.

Simmons-Martin, A.A., & Rossi, K.G. (1990). *Parents and teachers: Partners in language development.* Washington, DC: A.G Bell Association.

Simser, J. (1993). Auditory-verbal intervention: Infants and toddlers. *Volta Review, 95(3),* 217–229.

Simser, J. (1999). Parents: The essential partner in the habilitation of children with hearing impairment. *Australian Journal of Education of the Deaf, 5,* 55–62.

Smaldino, J.J., Crandall, C.C., Kreisman, B.M., John, A.B., & Kreisman, N.V. (2008). Room acoustics for listeners with normal hearing and hearing impairment. In M. Valente, H. Hosford-Dunn & R.J. Roeser (Eds.), *Audiology treatment (2nd ed.).* New York: Thieme, 418–451.

Smith, C.R. (1975). Residual hearing and speech production in deaf children. *Journal of Speech and Hearing Research, 18,* 795–811.

Spencer, P.E., & Marschark, M. (2003). Cochlear implants: Issues and implications. In M. Marschark & P.E. Spencer (Eds.), *Oxford handbook of deaf studies, language, and education.* New York, NY: Oxford University Press, 434–448.

Srinivasan, P. (1996). *Practical aural rehabilitation for speech-language pathologists and educators of hearing-impaired children.* Springfield, IL: Thomas.

Stackhouse, J., & Wells, B. (1997). *Children's speech and literacy difficulties: A psycholinguistic approach.* London: Whurr.

Stapells, D.R. (2000). Threshold estimation by the tone-evoked auditory brainstem response: A literature meta-analysis. *Journal of Speech-Language Pathology and Audiology, 24*, 74–83.

Stoker, R.G., & French-St. George, M. (1987). Effects of short-term training on the lipreadability of speakers. Paper presented at the Convention of the American Speech-Language Hearing Association, New Orleans, LA.

Stredler-Brown, A. (2010). Development of listening and language skills in children who are deaf or hard of hearing. In R.H. Hull (Ed.), *Introduction to aural rehabilitation*. San Diego, CA: Plural.

Streng, A., Fitch, W.J., Hedgecock, L.D., Phillips, J.W., & Carrell, J.A. (1955). *Hearing therapy for children*. New York: Grune & Stratton.

Sumby, W.H., & Pollack, I. (1954). Visual contribution to speech intelligibility in noise. *Journal of the Acoustical Society of America, 26*, 212–215.

Summerfield, Q. (1987). Speech perception in normal and impaired hearing. *British Medical Bulletin, 43*, 909–925.

Summers, I.R. (Ed.) (1992). *Tactile aids for the hearing impaired*. London: Whurr.

Tait, M., Nikolopoulos, T.P., Archbold, S., & O'Donoghue, G.M. (2001). Use of the telephone in prelingually deaf children with a multichannel cochlear implant. *Otology and Neurotology, 22(1)*, 47–52.

Tait, M.E., Nikolopoulos, T.P., & Lutman, M.E. (2007). Age at implantation and development of vocal and auditory preverbal skills in implanted deaf children. *International Journal of Pediatric Otorhinolaryngology, 71*, 603–610.

Thompson, S.C. (2002). Microphone, telecoil, and receiver options: Past, present, and future. In M. Valente (Ed.), *Hearing aids: Standards, options, and limitations (2nd ed.)*. New York, NY: Thieme, 64–100.

Tobey, E.A., Geers, A.E., & Brenner, C. (1994). Speech production results: Speech feature acquisition. *Volta Review, 96, 5 (monograph)*, 109–129.

Tobey, E.A., Geers, A.E., Brenner, C., Altuna, D., & Gabbert, G. (2003). Factors associated with development of speech production skills in children implanted by age five. *Ear and Hearing, 24*, 36S–45S.

Tomblin, J.B., Peng, S-C, Spencer, L. J., & Lu, N. (2008). Long-term trajectories of the development of speech sound production in pediatric cochlear implant recipients. *Journal of Speech, Language, and Hearing Research, 51*, 1353–1368.

Tye-Murray, N. (1994). *Let's converse: A "How-to" guide to develop and expand conversational skills of children and teenagers who are hearing impaired*. Washington, DC: A.G. Bell Association.

Tye-Murray, N. (2003). Conversational fluency of children who use cochlear implants. *Ear and Hearing, 24 (Suppl.)*, 82S–89S.

Tye-Murray, N., & Schum, L. (1994). Conversation training for frequent communication partners. In J-P Gagné & N. Tye-Murray (Eds.), Research in audiological rehabilitation: Current trends and future directions. *Journal of the Academy of Rehabilitative Audiology, 27 (Suppl)*, 209–222.

Tye-Murray, N., Spencer, L., & Gilbert-Bedia, E. (1995a). Relationships between speech production and speech perception skills in young cochlear-implant users. *Journal of the Acoustical Society of America, 98*, 2454–2460.

Tye-Murray, N., Spencer, L., & Woodworth, G.G. (1995b). Acquisition of speech by children who have prolonged cochlear implant experience. *Journal of Speech and Hearing Research, 38*, 327–337.

Uchanski, R.M. (2005). Clear speech. In D.B. Pisoni & R.E. Remez (Eds.), *The handbook of speech perception*. Malden, MA: Blackwell, 207–235.

REFERENCES

Uchanski, R.M., & Geers, A.E. (2003). Acoustic characteristics of the speech of young cochlear implant users: A comparison with normal-hearing age-mates. *Ear and Hearing, 24*, 90S–105S.

Urbantschitsch, V. (1895). *Auditory training for deaf mutism and acquired deafness.* [English trans. by S.R. Silverman, 1985]. Washington, DC: A.G. Bell Association for the Deaf.

Valimaa, T.T., Maatta, T.K., Lopponen, H.J., & Sorri, M.J. (2002a). Phoneme recognition and confusions with multichannel cochlear implants: Vowels. *Journal of Speech, Language, and Hearing Research, 45*, 1039–1054.

Valimaa, T.T., Maatta, T.K., Lopponen, H.J., & Sorri, M.J. (2002b). Phoneme recognition and confusions with multichannel cochlear implants: Consonants. *Journal of Speech, Language, and Hearing Research, 45*, 1055–1069.

van Uden, A. (1970). *A world of language for deaf children.* Rotterdam, NL: Rotterdam University Press.

van Uden, A. (1977). *A world of language for deaf children (3rd ed.).* Amsterdam: Swets & Zeitlinger.

Vermeulen, A.M., Snik, A.F.M., Brokx, J.P.L., van den Broek, P., Geelen, C.P.L., & Beijk, C.M. (1997). Comparison of speech perception performance in children using a cochlear implant with children using hearing aids based on the concept of "equivalent hearing loss". *Scandinavian Audiology, 47 (Suppl.)*, 55–57.

Walden, B.E., Prosek, R.A., Montgomery, A.A., Scherr, C.K., & Jones, C.J. (1977). Effects of training on the visual recognition of consonants. *Journal of Speech and Hearing Research, 20*, 130–145.

Wardhaugh, R. (1985). *How conversation works.* Oxford: Blackwell.

Watson, L.M., & Gregory, S. (2005). Non-use of cochlear implants in children: Child and parent perspectives. *Deafness and Education International, 7*, 43–58.

Watzlawick, P., Bavelas, J.B., & Jackson, D.D. (1967). *Pragmatics of human communication: A study of interactional patterns, pathologies, and paradoxes.* New York: Norton.

Wedenberg, E. (1951). Auditory training for deaf and hard of hearing children. *Acta Oto-Laryngologica, 39, (Suppl. 94)*.

Wedenberg, E. (1954). Auditory training of severely hard of hearing preschool children. *Acta Oto-Laryngologica, 44, (Suppl. 110)*.

Weiner, S., & Goodenough, D. (1977). A move toward a psychology of conversation. In R. Freedle (Ed.), *Discourse production and comprehension*, Norwood, NJ: Ablex, 213–225.

Weisenberger, J.M., & Percy, M.E. (1994). Use of the Tactaid II and Tactaid VII with children. *Volta Review, 96 (5, monograph)*, 41–57.

Whitehead, R.L. (1983). Some respiratory and aerodynamic patterns in the speech of the hearing impaired. In I. Hochberg, H. Levitt & M.J. Osberger (Eds.), *Speech of the hearing impaired: Research, training, and personnel preparation.* Baltimore, MD: University Park Press, 97–116.

Woodhouse, L., Hickson, L., & Dodd, B. (2008). Review of visual speech perception by hearing and hearing-impaired people: Clinical implications. *International Journal of Language and Communication Disorders, 25*, 1–18.

Yoshinaga-Itano, C. (1998). Development of audition and speech: Implications for early intervention with infants who are deaf or hard-of-hearing. In C. Yoshinaga-Itano & A. Sedey (Eds.), Language, speech, and social-emotional development of children who are deaf or hard-of-hearing: The early years. *Volta Review, 100 (5, monograph)*, 213–234.

Yule, G. (1997). *Referential communication tasks.* Mahwah, NJ: Erlbaum.

Zeiser, M.L., & Erber, N.P. (1977). Auditory/vibratory perception of syllabic structure in words by profoundly hearing-impaired children. *Journal of Speech and Hearing Research, 20*, 430–436.

Index

Related products developed by the author

HELOS hearing-loss simulator software

This software is used to modify the sound qualities of speech so that a person with normal hearing can experience what a hearing-impaired child perceives. Educators and audiologists use HELOS to create recorded demonstrations and to implement live, interactive communication training.

Available from Helosonics (Australia). **www.hearingvision.com**

QUEST?AR communication practice

This activity provides a framework for conversation and promotes the use of clarification strategies. The child asks a series of questions and listens to the adult's answers. Vocabulary and language are chosen to match the child's skill level. The QUEST?AR kit includes a booklet, list of topics, applications, and strategies.

Available from Helosonics (Australia). **www.hearingvision.com**

DYALOG communication analysis software

This software helps a teacher or therapist describe a child's conversational performance. The computer's space bar is pressed during intervals of conversational breakdown and repair. The result is a DYALOG summary graph and four quantitative measures that are components of conversational fluency.

Available from Parrot Software (USA). **www.parrotsoftware.com**